MEDICALLY SPEAKING,

WHO CONNECTS YOUR DOTS?

A Guide to Critical Thinking

Jill Fandrich, PharmD

ISBN 979-8-88851-728-4 (Paperback)
ISBN 979-8-88851-730-7 (Hardcover)
ISBN 979-8-88851-729-1 (Digital)

Covenant Books
11661 Hwy 707
Murrells Inlet, SC 29576
www.covenantbooks.com

CONTENTS

INTRODUCTION FOR *MEDICALLY SPEAKING, WHO CONNECTS YOUR DOTS?*

How do you interpret *medical* information? How do you digest the content you absorb from news sources today? Were you there to verify the facts? What about information presented online or in a book? How do you know if the information is *really* true? Do you have any *inside* connections to verify the content? Or are you, like the rest of us, trying to find some way to "connect the dots"? What do you know about *critical thinking*?

One day I listened to a story from a particular news source. It was almost fascinating to witness how emotionally charged one reporter had been while delivering her message and how passionate she was that only *her* version of the story was the *right* one. She was even visibly upset with anyone who expressed an opposing view. I then selected an alternate station and watched a different reporter share the same story with similar heartfelt concern but from an opposing viewpoint, conveying *his* version as the only *accurate* one. He also became outwardly agitated at the sounds of someone opposing his view. Each reporter displayed zeal, just as comparably intensive as the other, and each was also deemed believable, yet they had clearly secured opposing positions. *How can this be?* Two separate stations, two different reporters, the same topic, yet completely opposing views, while both claimed to be factual. I repeated this process numerous times with random stations, and the results were consistent. There were opposing positions, and each one *passionately* professed to be the accurate one. So, *who is right?*

I will admit that there was a time before this when I chose a stance, almost simply because it was what I *wanted* to be the right story. I found myself caught up in the frenzy and emotion of it all, which was not hard to do! The eye-opener for me occurred as my firm, definitive, infallible, 100 percent right, no-way-can-it-ever-be-wrong stance was—well—*wrong*! I admit it was wrong. *I was wrong.* I was shell-shocked and had to *scramble* to get the "egg" off my face. I don't like to be wrong. I don't think anyone *likes* to be wrong. Once I finally acknowledged my error, I asked myself, *Now what?*

Being analytical, my first line of action was to bring myself to an awareness of what was happening around me. I took a step back to collect information and assess the situation. What essentially happened was that I began to think critically about what was occurring "out there" in society, especially regarding *medical* information. This led me to ask question after question, seeking to find honest, substantial answers. I realized that the only "logical" answer lies in the ability to *think critically* about everything of importance.

A lack of *proper* thinking appears to have crept into our society. As mentioned, I have personally experienced this, which has shown me the need to bring forth a book such as this. What if you could begin to listen to any source of news, hear what is being said without a preconceived bias, and consider the information without becoming emotionally charged or passionate about being "right"? Then listen to an opposing view with the same unprejudiced stature, all *before* formulating an opinion or drawing a conclusion.

Whatever your reasons are for seeking additional information, this book will give you the tools and insight needed to significantly improve your ability to decipher medical content without emotion, discern truth from "nontruth" with confidence and candor, and increase your ability to handle any situation with a logically based conclusion. Critical thinking is a means to expand the *way* you think, open your mind to new thoughts and perspectives, increase the probability of uncovering factual information, and reduce the volatile impact fed from news media outlets.

I have discovered a need to return to the basics of *thought processing.* The most challenging problem that we all face, quite possibly, is dealing with the people around us—whether within your work setting, organizations, patient connections, networks, or even your home. There is always a need to develop the finesse, compassion, and especially the fine art of "getting along" with other people in everyday interactions.

In preparation for writing this book, I studied news sources and observed actions and reactions. I read numerous articles, studies, trials, and books and even attended an in-depth study regarding critical thinking, human behavior, and responses. I questioned rational professionals and not-so-sensical ones as well. With each topic, I visualized situations relevant to each one and how they could be applied to professional and personal settings. I also extrapolated critical findings from my experience in both my medical profession and intimate encounters. I organized the information in such a way that would be applicable from numerous perspectives. When applied, these skills and strategies will always prove to be practical, insightful, and *thought-altering*.

Relationships are the most essential things in our lives. It is logical to focus a significant amount of time and energy on understanding the nature of people, including our patients, and how our actions affect them. It should be an instinct to show love, kindness, and compassion in every interaction that occurs throughout our days, no matter whom we may come into contact with. Notice, I didn't say it would be easy! It is essential to display *tolerance* as you listen to opposing views and value the *person*, even if you disagree with their content. Learn how *not* to be sensitized by a different perspective. Just as important as it is to have finesse and charisma in our interactions, we must also display the qualities of compassion and tolerance in the *physical* actions we perform as well.

This book is interactive and meant to *educate*, *inform*, and *instruct*. Within each chapter, you will be brought to an awareness of certain content; then, you will be challenged to actively participate as you gradually yet consistently develop critical thinking skills. This book explores skills that will refine you as a logical thinker and decision-maker. We look at admirable qualities that will set you apart, illuminate your current skills, and allow you to justify a position as a rational thinker. Read or listen to each section slowly and deliberately, yet with vigor and passion, while underlining, highlighting, and jotting down notes about key points you want to incorporate into your thought processes and improve your skills. While trying these suggestions in every interaction may not be applicable, read or listen repeatedly to each section to program the information into your mind. Hence, you can access these *files* when the opportunity presents itself. Return and refer to these pages frequently, and even visualize the suggestions playing out in your own setting. Think about them often, and imagine different outcomes each time.

> Ask yourself the following:
> *How could I have applied critical thinking to my interactions today?*
> *What mistakes did I make?*
> *How can I do it differently next time?*
> *Where could I improve?*
> *What did I do right?*
> *What have I learned from this experience?*

Journal your results, whether they are "in progress" or are already successes. Be sure to enter the dates of each entry, and be specific regarding the interaction—what questions you asked, how you researched and collected data, and how you reached a *logical* decision. Include what you did or did not like about your interaction. For your convenience, there is an example "Journal" section at the back of this book, and a list of suggested *critical thinking questions*. Each may be replicated for your convenience. Review your journal weekly during the first year. Monitor your progress at least once a month to reveal how you are growing, and form a lifelong habit of logical thinking, personally and medically.

To understand the dire need to train your mind to think this way, you will also be introduced to definitions, trials, acts, applicable books paralleling current circumstances, and much more! By internalizing this information, you are sure to "imprint" inclusive thinking and successful traits into your mind's programming. While this is an enormous undertaking, learning about and genuinely understanding each chapter will undoubtedly grow you as a person and launch you as a decisive leader and clinician in your profession. Perhaps embrace one chapter per week and study it extensively. Understand what it means and the intent of the content and thoughts, methods, and reasons from the lists provided. Take time to answer the critical thinking questions listed. Visualize your own scenario with each query. Follow up with the concluding "Reflect" points at the end of each chapter. Spend time on each one, and decipher how you will incorporate this information into your professional, social, and personal life. You will begin to notice logical thinking being displayed more and more naturally in all of your interactions. Ask the same questions as previously mentioned, and journal how you turned emotionally charged information into a well-processed and logical conclusion, all while maintaining personal and professional relationships. Take the bias, emotions, and unwarranted opinions out of the situation. Finally, after the last chapter has been processed, go back to the beginning!

These methods will allow you to get the most out of this book. Whether you are a clinician in the medical profession, an administrator within an organization, head of your household, or an online medically inclined student, this book will masterfully remind you of the love, kindness, respect, compassion, *common sense, logic, sound reasoning*, and tolerance you should build into the very nature of your being and display throughout every interaction.

Let the process begin!

CHAPTER 1

Who Connects *Your* Dots?

What is meant by the words "*who connects your dots?*" Quite simply, who is *influencing* your thoughts, actions, responses, and methods of practicing? Do you have the freedom to make your own medical decisions based on your knowledge from past experience and study, or are you *told* what therapies or methods you are to employ? Who or what is the most medically influential *person* or *source* of information in your life? Do you draw upon content projected from the major news outlets, social media, Big Pharma, the Center for Disease Control and Prevention (CDC), medical journals, continuing education sources, or the Internet without question? Or do you consider the source, where it came from, whether or not bias is involved, what and whom it represents, and who is funding it, and then think for yourself?

There was a time when the media was "called out" and reprimanded if the stories they presented contained false implications to the slightest degree. Currently, however, there is no consequence for "misinformation." As a matter of fact, misinformation is now actually *approved and encouraged.* I'm unsure if you caught that or just skimmed over the last sentence. Yes, misinformation is now *permitted* in our media culture and has existed for quite some time.

How can you incorporate this piece of information into your analysis when evaluating information? It is imperative to now consider this. Most major news outlets are derived from the *same* common source, owned by the *same* company or proprietor, and produce and portray the *same* deceptive content, with the goal of infiltrating, manipulating, propagating, or even inculcating people with tainted data based on "their agenda" of what they want you to know, believe, think, and how to practice. If you work for a type of institution such as a hospital or someone else's establishment, who or what is the source of funding? *Follow the money.*

Knowing this, it is essential to bring yourself to an *awareness* of this very operation that is occurring. Begin to ask yourself questions. Who owns each of the news stations? Who owns Big Pharma? Who owns the medical journals? Who controls them? How does Big Pharma prosper from given situations? What information are they providing funding for? What is their common link or links? Where is the source of information coming from? Are they for-profit or non-profit? How might the message be skewed?

Understand that you were not actually on location to know if these events really occurred or if the words spoken or written carry any validity. Propaganda is *no longer* required to be truthful. You do not have any proof of the expressed content. You are being told what *they want* you to believe. Are you allowing *them* to "connect your dots" for you, and are you accepting what they say as true and accurate? Or will you listen with an open mind, consider the content and the source, *follow the money*, research other sources, and derive your own conclusions? How can you find out more information to substantiate the provided subject matter? Is it possible that there might be other versions of the story? Or could the story have possibly been altered to fit a scenario?

As a medically inclined person, you have a distinct and probably gifted ability to analyze information in depth and use logical reasoning to draw your own conclusions. However, have you been using this ability in your reasoning, especially within the past few years? Now that the media is *no longer required* to present true content as they share information, performing your own detailed and thorough critical analysis is imperative.

From the moment you were born, other people have been programming your mind with *their* opinions, viewpoints, processes, and slews of other information. Your parents or guardians who raised you have shared their version of information, which was embedded in your mind. You absorbed additional information from professors, friends, televisions, newspapers, media, social media, the Internet, books, journals, articles, reviews, studies, trials, and dozens of other third-party sources. Other than what you personally have experienced, all of this data input has been presented to you, often with little to no evidence or full disclosure of truth to support or substantiate it or perhaps with *inaccurate* information to "support" it.

How often do you actually think for yourself regarding what has been presented or claimed? Do you already realize that the multitude of your thoughts has been preprogrammed by other sources? Does this knowledge come as a surprise? Or did you understand this concept already? Are your automatic responses to situations in line with what you believe in? Do you even know *what* you believe in? What are your thoughts about *reprogramming* your mind to align with your values?

In what ways do you educate yourself? Do you just listen to continuing education from someone else's point of view and "assume" it is correct? How about articles or clinical studies? How "in-depth" do you pursue the information? What if they have been misinformed even if the intentions are honorable? Do you *assume* medical journals are correct without discovering their connections to Big Pharma, government agencies, or others who may have a financial or political agenda? Do you listen to the "worldview" and conform to what *they* think, say, and conclude? Do they have your personal and professional best interests at heart? Do these educational sources have the *patients'* best interests at heart? What financial incentive may be tied to the information? Who is funding the study or the content of the information?

Be particular about the sources of education, discover *who* wrote the books or journals or who is teaching the course, and know *what* they stand for and where their research stemmed from. Understand who backs them financially and who stands to prosper from the viewpoint they are presenting. It is becoming increasingly transparent that certain major and influential universities have taken an obvious and distinctive political stance rather than providing unbiased, factual, and historically objective educational content. Find out the basis for their viewpoint, how and why they select the particular content, and how their conclusions are derived. Who is funding them? What do they desire to achieve? Is unbiased information being presented to enhance the student? Or is there a biased and propagated agenda with the intention to persuade or manipulate? Is there an *expectation* that you *will* think like them, or else *you* are considered wrong and in violation, often with a penalty involved? Perhaps a grade or other incentive is related to whether or not you conform to their way of thinking.

It has become apparent that precious children have become the *ultimate source* and target for initiating change in this world. If society can program children with the thoughts and ideation *they* want to provoke, rather than relying on the teachings of home and family values, the culture will begin to be, in essence, "brainwashed" to think and respond in the same ways desired and designed by the society or the controlling governing body. Without realizing it, your ability to think freely and undefiled is gradually being compromised and quashed through various and even intricate modalities.

Can you see evidence of bias presented in the news sources? How about propaganda from Big Pharma? What appears to be the underlying theme? Observe *several different* and *opposing* stations if you can find them. Take some time to analyze your own thoughts regarding each content individually, the approach, and the viewpoint. Then, compare and contrast the similarities and differences you discovered through your analysis. You must take an *unbiased* stance, consider what is presented, and discover whether or not they are relaying facts or opinions or trying to persuade you to any degree.

What have you noticed? What is your go-to news source? Are you able to *objectively* watch different sources and uncover dramatically different vantage points and opinions of the same story or event? How about different medical sources of information? Take a step back and consider what you have revealed. Do any that you have observed present objective and factual stories from an unbiased perspective with the intent of informing you of proven objective details while allowing you to come to *your own* conclusion? Are the sources of the content *fully* revealed?

My point here is not to provoke you to pick one side over another and follow blindly but rather to consider both or all sides and realize how the intent is quite often to *manipulate* you into taking *a* side. You are an intelligent person. As a medical professional or someone who is medically inclined in some way, you undoubtedly have the ability to analytically think for yourself. You were born with a moral code and have an innate sense of right and wrong. You have the desire to help, to heal, and to *first do no harm* to people. Now more than ever in history, you are *losing* the very freedom and individuality your ancestors fought hard to provide.

Consider when you first started practicing in your field of expertise. What choices in treatment or therapy were you able to choose from? Was it actually *your* choice? And now, what percentage of the time are you currently instructed to treat in a certain mandated or formalized way? Are you banned from certain treatments you previously found safe and effective? How has this affected the way you treat your patients? How much of your freedom of practice has been lost? While it appeared to be gradual and subtle for decades, it is now *blatantly* apparent and exponentially driven that your freedom is being reframed with manipulation, brainwashing, herd mentality, and conformity, almost definitely derived from a stance of money, power, and control and *not* from a position of "patient care."

Ways your freedom is being purloined

1. *News media outlets.* It is quite difficult to deny that *nearly all* news sources are biased in one way or another. Understand that each one has *its* own agenda. Consider what that agenda may be and use your own moral code to interpret the content. Bias generally carries an intent to persuade, manipulate, deceive, or even brainwash. Research whom they are funded by. The media *no longer* follows a code of ethics in presenting true and unbiased facts. *Know this* as you read or listen to the content of *any* news source.

Understand that they are no longer held accountable for presenting the truth. Ask yourself, Who is presenting this information? Who owns the station? What seems to be the reason for this portrayal or vantage point? What appears to be the desired end result of the content? How or what could this change? Who will benefit from this viewpoint? Does the source appear to have an agenda? Does it appear to be ignoring, overlooking, or leaving out information in an attempt to sway the viewers? Is there any type of manipulative language attempting to persuade you to their viewpoint? Find a news source with an opposing view. Follow through the same questions and assessment without prejudice, also discovering who funds them. Are they censoring anyone with an opposing viewpoint? Carefully evaluate the information objectively and draw your own conclusions. Make a conscious effort to gather as much information as possible before jumping to any conclusions. If you just heard the news from a major news outlet and believed it as the truth, you did *not* think critically. What information collected from all sources is most important? Evaluate the information you collected. What do you think is going on?

2. *Removing your history*. History *is* what it is. What would the point be to ignore it and pretend it didn't happen? That will not change the fact that it actually *did* happen. It is important to know what happened in the past, no matter how painful or fascinating it may be, and to see how much we have grown as a country, continent, and world. Look at the immeasurable value of vast medical advancements attained through historical measures, knowledge, successes, and failures of the medical professionals before your time and how their discoveries have changed the course of medicine, time and again. You have the right and *privilege* of knowing the truth of your predecessors and how you have been shaped *because* of them. "Society" today is trying to erase the past and pretend it didn't happen or, worse yet, conceal the details from you, relinquishing it from your mind. It

is important to think about this fact and ask yourself why they would want to erase the knowledge of authentic past events from your mind. Deeply consider how you would benefit from having yet another thing hidden from your mind. How many "political" things are currently hidden from you already? Are you willing to give up more of your privileged rights? Who or what is the source instigating this movement? Who benefits from attempting to erase historical facts from your information base? What does it solve by pretending historical events did not happen? What seems to be the reason for erasing historical facts from your mind? What is the end result of burying this disclosure? Does it change the fact that it really *did* happen? *Why* are "they" intent on doing this? What information can you gather to shed more light on this subject? Where can you find unbiased data so you may extrapolate and discover your own conclusions?

3. *Educational content.* Education at all levels should be, and was, a means for filling your mind with facts and true events. The initial purpose was to grow in knowledge and gain a deeper understanding of how things work or operate, why things function the way they do, what actually happened, and so forth. The intent and, therefore, the content have changed from factual knowledge of your choosing to biased agendas of what "the system" wants you to believe. Why has society taken God out of public schools? Whom does this benefit? What appears to be the agenda for this? What about the information they are now presenting in general? Is it based on fact, or is it biased? Who is behind curriculum changes in the educational system? Are the clinical trials "cooked" in any way? Who funded the trials? Is the placebo claimed within the trials actually *"safety neutral,"* or are they using a *previous* drug or vaccine as the "placebo" and then claiming that the new drug has little variance in adverse effects compared to the placebo? Were they *truly* blinded if that is what was claimed? If education

or studies are biased in *any* way, they are no longer education; they are now propaganda. What colleges have shifted from education to propaganda? What might their agenda be? Who is funding the schools or educational platform? Is there a common link? Why was there a gradual and now progressive conformity in the chosen content? What seems to be the reason for these changes? What appears to be the desired end result? What will this change? Are they overlooking, ignoring, or leaving out information that doesn't support their agenda? Why might this be? Are they using unnecessary language or bias to sway the participants' perceptions of *their* ideas or beliefs? What might their reasoning be for their efforts to influence you into accepting their biasing of what should be factual and educational information? Where can you find unbiased resources so you may evaluate this information or use resources that are already there but look at them with fresh eyes and question the process? For example, review clinical studies and question the parameters, the labeling, the placebo used, and the like. Verify if it was blinded or not. How will you determine which sources are reliable, credible, and unbiased? What do you think is going on? Evaluate the information you collect and draw your own conclusions.

4. *Mandates.* Mandates are orders put in place by the authority of the one in a position to do so. What mandates are currently in effect in society today? What mandates have recently been in place in your area of practice? What mandates currently affect you? What is the ultimate source of the mandates? How did the source benefit from creating these mandates? Was there a financial incentive for the source? Have you taken time to *follow the money*? What scientific evidence have you reviewed regarding the mandates? Did you research what was being "mandated" before you followed through? What is the source of the evidence? Have you evaluated the reasons presented regarding the basis? Have you suddenly been "forced" to act, think, or

respond in certain ways based on certain information presented to you? What does the science tell you? Were you given access to unbiased resources to support the claim? Who has presented this information? What is the information upon which the mandates are based? Does the presenter have ties to a financial incentive in any way? Are there political ties? What seems to be the reason for the mandates? Has the information been presented in a way to "scare" you into doing something? Have *you* been offered a financial incentive to participate? What about a consequence if you do not? Does your facility have financial incentives for certain diagnoses or therapies? Has there been action by intimidation? What appears to be the end or desired result of the mandates? Whom do the mandates benefit? Does the source of the mandates appear to have an agenda? Is the source of the mandates overlooking, ignoring, or leaving out information that doesn't support the claims? Is there censorship or "shaming" if you do not conform and agree? Is any unnecessary information or language being used to sway your perception of the topic? Do the mandates interfere with any of your freedoms? Where can you find *unbiased research* from an ethical and trusted source to help understand the mandates? How will you verify the credibility of the research and the source? Once verified, infer and draw your own conclusions based on the information *you* gathered. Follow the true and *real science* from nonprofit sources and extrapolate your own logical results. What have you discovered? Did you reach this decision without prejudice or influence from any outside source?

5. *Entertainment industry.* Entertainment used to be lighthearted and enlightening, with the supposed intention of providing a pleasurable experience and some needed relaxation. It was an opportunity to let your mind drift from your current world and slip into the make-believe events of someone or something else. Today there is a deliber-

ate political message being portrayed and embedded in nearly all forms of entertainment, including movies, television shows, music, art, and even advertising in between. Subliminal messages are most likely "guaranteed" to be a part of the included exposure. Are you familiar with all the subliminal messages encapsulated throughout all forms of entertainment? Commercials and advertisements are now all about politics and propaganda. Their goal is to mesmerize and standardize *their* view and agenda and imprint it onto you, causing *you* to alter your way of reasoning, thinking, and believing. It is now a deliberate platform. What do you really know about subliminal messages? Where are subliminal messages hidden? What is their intent? Who benefits from them? How can you find out more about them? Why are people trying to influence you to *their* way of thinking and to "normalize" that which is not normal via commercials and entertainment content? In the entertainment realm, who is sending a political message? Who is funding it? What seems to be the reason for this message? Why have the majority of drug-related ads become driven to share a political message rather than present their product by unbiased means? Does the message have a bias? What appears to be the desired end result? How could this affect you? To whom does this message benefit? Does the source of the entertainment appear to have an agenda? Is the source ignoring, overlooking, or leaving out (censoring) information that doesn't support its beliefs? Is the source using provocative or other forms of biased language to sway the audience's perception? Maintain your own ability to think for yourself based on *your* own standards and beware of any intent to influence you and how you practice medicine. What information is being fed through all of the electronic devices held so dearly by hands, both large and small? Who controls these devices? Are they secretly invasive in your home or at the office? What are these devices capable of? Do they "seek" to collect personal information, practice information, or preferences about you? Do they display ads and persuasion without your direct permission, or even knowledge, for that matter? Where can you find unbiased and accurate information regarding all of this? What sources will you use in your research? How will you verify their credibility? What information is most relevant? Objectively analyze and evaluate this information and draw your own unprejudiced conclusions. What do you think is going on?

6. *Big Pharma and medicine.* Big Pharma has become a powerful entity of its own. You must do your own independent research to find out details about when, why, who they really are, and who controls them. My goal is simply to bring awareness to this growing enigma, not define the precise composition. A large conglomerate of drug sources and individual proprietors, and then some, comprise this entity of powerful control. Research and find out more about Big Pharma, who specifically controls them, who "owns" them, who funds them, how powerful they have become, and how they profit from their involvement in the most recent mandates, among other things. There was a time when virtually the only source of drug advertising consisted of drug representatives propagating their product, attempting to influence physicians, pharmacists, and other medical personnel, with the intention of having their items chosen for a preferred drug formulary. Nowadays, drug advertising is not only in every venue but also contains an inflamed sociopolitical agenda, more powerful than you can even imagine. To make a logical and informed decision regarding your choices and conclusions, ask yourself many fact-seeking questions. Who is propagating the particular drug, vaccine, or other mechanisms? Who is funding the propagation? Who is funding the clinical trials or research? Is there a politically charged message attached? What are they proposing? What seems to be the reason for doing this? How can you verify safety and efficacy? What appears

to be the desired end result? How could this change things? Who would benefit from this product being chosen for use or consumption? Who would benefit from the sale of this product? How long has the product been on the market? What type of research was performed on it before it reached the market? Did it go through proper clinical trials? How can you verify that? Do they reveal what was used as the placebo, if one was used at all? Was it "safety neutral," such as saline, or was it a previous version of the vaccine or drug so they could claim that it had a *similar adverse effect*" profile? Has it been used for any other indication through the years? Have any medications that have been safely used for years suddenly been deemed "unsafe," not based on any new results or side effects, but rather, "just because"? How many years has it been safely used, and what type of research was performed regarding the product? Did new drugs or vaccines go through *all* of the proper steps of research and studies? Were the clinical trials "rushed" and cut short, bypassing normal safety and efficacy studies? Were there studies actually performed on *subpopulations* before deeming them safe for these categories? Would you prescribe, administer, or dispense a product to this category if they *weren't* performed? Were the studies blinded? What evidence is there to support this? What is the premise of this product? Are there other products similar to it? What makes one better than the other? What other choices do you have? Does the source of the product appear to have an agenda? Is the source using unnecessary verbiage with the intent of swaying the perception of the consumer? How are medical staff being persuaded to utilize the product? Are they being "threatened" to use the product, leaving them with a penalty if they don't? Are both sides of the story being presented, or just one side with the intent to persuade? Is there any censorship if someone presents with a differing vantage point? Are there incentives for its usage? Are there penalties if it's not used? Are hospitals receiving "kickbacks" for certain drug use or even diagnoses? How can you find out this information? What reactions have occurred since the inception of the product? *Follow the money* and discover who receives monetary benefits in the medical domain. The ability to infer is vital in order to draw logical conclusions based on your findings. Where can you find untainted information? How will you verify your resources? What information is relevant for discovery to draw your conclusions? Assess the information based on unbiased raw data and extrapolate potential outcomes. What do you think is going on?

7. *Social media.* Social media has taken the world by storm. Few, if any, cultures are not impacted by this form of communication. A choice can be made whether to use this device positively or negatively, to affect, inform, or influence others. That is in the eye and decision of the beholder. Along with the favorable ability to connect with long-lost family, friends, or other people, social media has also become an unfavorable method of propagation and political influence. Who has devised the message? What seems to be the reason for this message? Is there a reason behind the timing of the message? What appears to be the desired end result of the message? How could this affect you? Who could be mainly affected? To whom does this message benefit? Does the source of this message appear to have an agenda? Are there monetary rewards involved? Is the source of the message overlooking, ignoring, or leaving out pertinent information that doesn't support the beliefs or claim? Is there censorship to anyone with an opposing view? If so, why would that be? What are the reasons someone would censor someone else? Does the source use particular verbiage or type of language to influence the reader or listener? Is there emotion built into the message? Is there an intent to instill fear in the viewer? Attempt to gather information from opposing viewpoints. Do not allow your personal biases to cloud your judgment. If you approach the

research with a bias of any kind, you are *no longer* critically thinking. How can you independently verify the information? Research the content and source, collecting as much raw data as possible. Use logic to evaluate the information. Identify evidence that forms *your* beliefs. Draw your own individual conclusions. What do you think is going on?

8. *Church and "religion."* There is a distinct difference between your belief and a "religion." While a belief is a mental conviction of truth and a church is a body of believers, a "religion" is a man-made title with rituals or "works" to be performed to gain approval. As mentioned previously, perform your own research for detail and clarity. This section is meant to bring awareness to this particular topic. Propaganda and false prophets have been slipping into the church for centuries. It continues today in even bigger and more obvious ways, although some ways are even more devious. This brings about the absolute need to evaluate information and engage in the process of critical thinking. Who is presenting the message? What seems to be the reason for the message? What is the desired end result of the message? Who is the message intended to glorify? How are you impacted by the message? Does it glorify an individual, a business, a fake idol, or a ritual, or does it glorify the Creator? How are you impacted by the message? In what ways are you impacted? Who benefits from the message? Is there a financial incentive behind the message? Is there any political funding involved? Does the source of the message appear to have an agenda? Is the source overlooking, ignoring, or leaving out information that doesn't support its beliefs or claims? Is the source using language meant to sway the parishioners' perception of the facts? What information is relevant to determine the answers? Where can you find unbiased information? Research this data from an unprejudiced perspective. Evaluate and analyze the information, and ask yourself again, *who* is the focus of the *glory*

of the message? Formulate your own conclusions. What has the information led you to discover?

9. *Politics.* Politics. Oh my, politics. What can be said about politics? I believe "politics" was intended to be "for the people." The people were to elect officials who promised to work hard and *serve the people.* The *people* were supposed to be the ones in control, not the government. It couldn't be further from this concept now. The political arena has become the center of self-serving agendas and a hub of propaganda. Thank goodness this is not the case with every elected official. However, it is the majority. That being said, it is important to do your own research and decide for yourself the meaning and intention of political actions and agendas. Who is doing a certain action? What are they doing? What seems to be the reason for this action? Why is it happening now? What are the intended end results of the action? How could this affect you? How could this affect your patients? Whom does this action benefit? Is there a monetary reward behind, or for, this action? Does the source of the action appear to have an agenda? Can you decipher what the agenda is? Is the source overlooking, ignoring, or leaving out information that doesn't support the beliefs or claims of the action? Is there censorship if someone presents with a differing viewpoint? Is the source of the action using persuasive language to sway the people's perception of a fact? Is there an intent to instill fear or intimidation in the people? Look at the opposing side of the source of action. Ask the same questions from an opposing perspective. Where do you find biases? What supports either view? How does this benefit either side? Is there an emotional reaction if someone chooses an opposing view to the one presented? Or is there freedom to think differently? Independently research and verify the information discovered. What sources will you use? How will you deem them reliable? What information is relevant for clarity? Evaluate the claims of opposing sides, keeping in

mind potential biases. Allow yourself to see things from both perspectives. Draw a logical conclusion based on your findings. What did you discover? *Follow the money.*

10. *Legal system.* The legal system is tied completely to the political system, being a branch of it. Some officials of the court are elected, and some are not. The people elect some, and some are elected by the people we elected. Your own research will provide more clarity to these words. For the same reasons mentioned previously, it is important to ask critical thinking questions regarding specifics in the legal system. Make yourself aware of potential bias, who elected the people into these positions, and the underlying reasons, such as financial, reputational, or even positional pressure. If there is censorship, ask yourself why. Always seek to find out who may be funding a person or event that may be occurring. Evaluate unbiased information you obtained through your own research. What do you conclude?

11. *Science and research.* Science *is* knowledge. It's a body of *facts* learned through study, observation, or experience. Generally, if you want to find the truth regarding something material or organic, you follow the science. *However,* even scientific *documentation* can be fabricated or manipulated by a human source. This again leads to the vital process of thinking critically. Regarding a new so-called vaccine or a suspicious virus, rather than make assumptions or engage in a "herd mentality," do *your own* research. Was the virus actually around years before it was said to have caused harm? Is the vaccine really a "vaccine" at all? Is the vaccine more harmful than the virus itself? Follow unbiased and true science. If someone or something is concealing evidence or will not reveal a source, it is important to ask yourself *why.* Who is making a scientific claim? What is the claim? What scientific evidence have you observed regarding the claim? How have you verified the validity of the scientific evidence? What seems to be the reason for the claim? Are they offering full disclosure? What appears to

be the end result of the claim? How could this affect you? How does this affect them? To whom does this claim benefit? Is anyone being censored if they propose a differing view? Why would there be censorship "if" everything was legitimate? *Follow the money.* Are there monetary benefits for this claim? Are there monetary benefits based on a volume of people conceding to this claim? Does the source of the claim appear to have an agenda in regard to it? Are there any other possible agendas involved? Is the source overlooking, ignoring, or *leaving out information* that doesn't support the claim? Is there any unnecessary or persuasive language used to sway the perception of the end user of the claim? Is there intimidation involved in promoting the product? How about fear? Is there an intention meant to create fear in people? Where can you find information about sources not biased toward this claim? Research many *unbiased* sources as you seek answers and factual knowledge. Where are you collecting the information from? Observe information from opposing sides of the claim. Is the research itself credible? Evaluate each side without prejudice. Are *you* reluctant to view the information from both sides of the claims? If so, why? Do you become emotionally charged or defensive if presented with opposing information? Determine the relevance of the information and focus on what is most important regarding the claim. Verify that the sources are credible. How will you determine if they are credible? Who is funding the research you are examining? What would allow you to put something into your body without verifying facts regarding the ingredients and their long-term effects? Would fear allow you to do this? What have you researched before allowing this to happen? Would you lay down your life on the guarantee to your trusting patients that the product you agree to dispense or inject into them will not harm them? What proof have you personally gathered? Know what goes into your body. Know what you are advocating to go into your patients' bodies. Are you willing to risk losing your license by only adhering to one side of the story provided? Assess all of the information you gathered and analyze the data. Draw your own conclusions based on *your* research. Where does it take you? What conclusions do you arrive at?

12. *Literature.* Literature can be entertaining, informative, educational, persuasive, humorous, sad, and so forth. It can be almost anything. Writing has been a part of society for thousands of generations as a way of communicating, educating, and preserving thoughts and ideas. Unfortunately, literature can also be deceptive. There is no requirement to relay true, honest, accurate, and completely factual content. So once again, it is important to ask many questions and consider the research you have personally collected regarding the literature and the source. Who is the author? What did they write? What are their backgrounds and qualifications? What seems to be the reason for writing the material? What appears to be the desired result of the material? Is there a benefit if they persuade you? How could this affect you? How could it affect the author? Whom does it benefit? Does the author appear to have an agenda? Are you able to identify the agenda? How about a political agenda? Is the author overlooking, ignoring, or leaving out information that may be contrary to the intended claim? Does the author use persuasive language to sway the readers' perception? Is there strong emotion, or any emotion, tied to the material? If it poses an argument, what can you learn about the opposing view? Does the author want you to avoid opposing information? How can you verify the facts or content within the material? Are they truthful? What unbiased sources can you use to find out more information? How will you verify the sources? Is the material meant for pleasure, to inform, or to persuade? Does the author reveal sources used for the material? Collect as much information as possible from credible sources. Evaluate the information objectively and draw your own conclusions. What did you

discover about the material? What about the author? What conclusions have you reached?

13. *Family, friends, or associates.* People you associate with can be *very* influential and opinionated for numerous reasons. Perhaps you are fond of them, loyal, curious, indebted, opposed, or maybe even intimidated by them. It is not always easy to know the motive behind what people do or say or even why. It is important to be able to decipher the validity of the person and any motives or intentions they may have, especially regarding you. Sometimes there is controversy within your own family unit. Perhaps it is with a coworker in your business setting. Lately, it may even be derived from a politically different standpoint. Be able to identify the necessity to evaluate them as well. What is it that they are doing or asking of you? What seems to be the reason for this? What appears to be the desired end result? How would this affect you? How would it affect them? Who does this action or request benefit? Do they appear to have an agenda? Are you able to identify the agenda? Are they overlooking, ignoring, or leaving out information contrary to their desire? Are they using persuasive, or even deceptive, language? Are they showing emotion or being defensive in their request? Are they using manipulative tactics? Is there some way to challenge their view with an opposing viewpoint? What information can you draw from this? What questions can you ask them to gain more understanding of the situation? How can you become fully aware of the basis of the request? Ask yourself questions, and critically think about the information you gathered. What conclusions have you reached based on the information?

This is just the tip of the iceberg. There are many additional ways in which your freedom is slipping away. Recall the massive iceberg that is said to have taken down the *Titanic*. According to the story presented, the majority of it dwelled hidden in the depths of the same icy, dark waters it rested upon, yet was capable of enormous devastation against many odds. Just as icebergs are deceiving, it is also possible for the information to be obscured or even deluded from the sphere of content made available to you while a multitude of hidden agendas lies beneath the surface.

As a medical person, you are designed to be analytical by nature. Yet, even as I recall my own training, there was never a course that explained or even encouraged critical thinking. Now more than ever, clinicians need to equip themselves with the ability to use logic and sound reasoning for drawing conclusions in a world now driven by propagation and manipulation. Big Pharma is about money, control, and power rather than being patient-centered and person-oriented. It is important to understand and acknowledge this awareness. Do extensive research on your own and *follow the money*. Seek to understand their position in the government and the world. Find out who owns them, controls them, and benefits from their success. Find unbiased and opposing sources of research and then collect the data and evaluate them for yourself. Recall your reasons for pursuing your field of expertise in the first place, and always abide by your oath to *first do no harm* to another person.

Patients have entrusted their precious lives into your capable hands. Is your research from major media outlets, for-profit medical journals, or for-profit, government-owned, or influenced drug companies (Big Pharma)? Or did your research come from scientists who gain nothing from sharing their nonprofit research in the name of science and patient care? Find out more and train yourself to start thinking critically in your realm of practice. As the medical field has always been considered a trusted field, built upon caring, compassionate, and passionate individuals, there is also a tendency to "go with the flow" and believe what is being revealed from sources that are *expected* to be credible. I challenge you to remain caring, compassionate, and passionate, yet begin to ask questions and seek information from opposing views while remaining unbiased without any preconceived answers. If you find yourself emotionally charged regarding this challenge or resistant to do this, again, *ask yourself why* you would rather "feel" that you were "right" rather than be open to discovering more information. Question the research and challenge its validity. Know when it's time to pick your battles and dig a little deeper rather than take things at face value. You can't go wrong by discovering more. Evaluate *all* information collected before drawing *your own* conclusions. What have you discovered?

The only freedom that is of enduring importance is the freedom of intelligence, that is to say, freedom of observation and of judgment, exercised on behalf of purposes that are intrinsically worthwhile. The commonest mistake made about freedom is, I think, to identify it with freedom of movement, or, with the external or physical side of activity.
—John Dewey

If you are influenced to think the way others think without first thinking for yourself, are you really free?
—Jill Fandrich

The most effective way to destroy people is to deny and obliterate their own understanding of their history.
—George Orwell

You can sway a thousand men by appealing to their prejudices quicker than you can convince one man by logic.
—Robert A. Heinlein

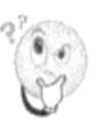

Reflect

1. Who is connecting your dots? Do you question the validity of medical resources and even challenge the extent of the research they claim? What changes will you make as a result of this chapter's revelation?

2. Watch different news sources (with different owners) and listen to both sides of the same story. What is the basis for each opposing view?

3. Question the social media content when politically inclined, and research facts about the topic at hand before formulating an opinion. What is an opposing viewpoint? What have you discovered?

4. Do you allow yourself to take the viewpoint of whoever is presenting the information first? How can you gain more control over your own thoughts and actions without persuasion from others?

5. Define your moral code by which you evaluate incoming information, especially medical information. Use this basis to ask questions when presented with information.

6. How do you choose educational sources for yourself and your patients and customers? Where do you research for the basis of the content? How can you verify the intent of the content? Is there any bias?

7. Identify your core values and incorporate them into your mind's programming.

8. What do you do to protect yourself from conformity?

9. Identify the ways your freedom is being purloined. What other ways can you think of in which freedom is slipping away from you?

10. How do you handle medical information presented to you? Do you automatically believe the content? Do you research the source, and who benefits from this information? How can you critically think about medical information presented to you? Who is funding the research? Remember to *follow the money.*

CHAPTER 2

What Is Critical Thinking?

What exactly *is* critical thinking? It is the ability to observe and think about a situation and to see and assess its validity or reality based on *your own* research and analysis without outside influence or bias. *"Critical thinking is the analysis of an issue or situation and the facts, data or evidence related to it."*[1] You take time to see the essential truth based on logic and common sense. You "challenge" what has been said or shown and consider numerous possible answers or alternatives. The key is to ask questions wherever possible. Never stop asking questions. This is to be performed objectively without influence from personal feelings, opinions, peers, or biases. The focus should be entirely based on factual information. Perhaps even discover new ways of thinking about things. You must be able to do this without being biased or prejudiced. Where is the evidence of proof? What is the source of evidence? Who is involved? Are they reliable? How can you verify their credibility? You have been blessed with tremendous brain power and the capacity to think critically. Use this ability to think with an open mind and consider the validity of the presented information.

Critical thinking is a skill that can be practiced and mastered. It allows you to make logical and informed decisions to the best of your abilities. There is no particular standard for how critical thinking occurs, and numerous approaches exist. However, some basic concepts that can guide you to becoming an exceptional critical thinker will be presented. It is important to *identify what is occurring*. What is the situation or problem at hand, and what factors may be influencing it? Gain clarity of the situation, including who and what may be influential. Ask questions such as *Who is doing what? What seems to be the reason for this happening?* and *What are the end results, and how could they change?*

The next step is to undergo intensive and independent *research*, comparing arguments about the issue of concern from opposing vantage points. Arguments are persuasive and influential. Therefore, it is important that your research be performed *independently* by you and that the resources be verified as factual, reliable, credible, and unbiased. Evaluate the research and resources from both sides. Are the claims that are made "sourced" or "unsourced"? If the claims do not have a specified source, or you discover they are seeking to "hide" the source, that is a red flag, leading to the question of *why?* Continue to research this *new* question and add the data to the other collected information.

It is important to be aware that the presented information may not be as it "seems." For example, a study may claim to use a placebo as a control. Yet if you dig deeper, you may find it was *not* a "neutral" control, as in *all* vaccinations currently approved for the standard children's series of vaccinations presently given. *Not one* of them used a *pure neutral* placebo compared to the vaccine itself.[2] This way, the claim could be made that the adverse effects weren't *significantly different* from the placebo.

Biases are sometimes very difficult to uncover, yet this is vital to the critical thinking process. The most skilled critical thinkers seek to master this difficult ability. Strong critical thinkers do their best to evaluate information objectively and view the claims of *both* sides of an argument. It is important to be able to wade through the waters of biases that likely are included on both sides. While *identifying biases*, it is equally important to set aside your own biases to ensure your judgment does not become clouded.

Try challenging yourself to debate one side of the argument, justifying it until you win the argument. Then, do *the same thing* for the opposing side of the argument! What have you learned from this exercise? Learn to see things from different vantage points and be objective in doing so. Analyze the evidence that forms your own beliefs and verify that the sources are credible and reliable. Questions to ask when evaluating bias include the following: *Whom does this benefit? Does the source of this information appear to have an agenda? Is the source overlooking, ignoring, or leaving out information that doesn't support its beliefs or claims?* and *Is this source using unnecessary language to sway an audience's perception of a fact? Who is funding "the source"?* Also, identify if there is censorship involved. If so, ask yourself, *if* the information "the source" is presenting is sound and truthful, *why* would there be paranoia leading to censoring? Censoring is a *defensive* stance driven by insecurity. There should *always* be a red flag when censoring is identified. More on censorship is included in a future chapter.

Next, it is important to use *logical reasoning* and draw conclusions based on the sound evidence you gathered. To master the skill of critical thinking, it is important to be able to *infer* and create an *educated* "guess" based on your thorough research. You must extrapolate and discover potential outcomes based on the raw data collected. Assess the information and draw your own conclusions. As not all inferences will be correct, it becomes crucial to make a conscious effort to gather as much untainted information as possible before reaching this decision.

It can also be challenging, yet important, to *discern the relevance* of the information for your consideration and seek the *most relevant* data. There may be a multitude of data out there regarding the topic, and you must decipher what is most pertinent to reaching your desired direction. What is your end goal? Determine precisely what it is you desire to uncover or discover.

Finally, be open to *unbiased discovery* by asking open-ended questions. This allows all possibilities without prejudice. Information that is unfiltered and unprompted may be revealed by asking questions in this format. A free flow of information is encouraged, and there is a greater potential that productive information may be produced that may further guide your evaluation of data.

Research and find additional ways to perform the skill of critical thinking. While there are many methods to implore this process, we discussed the need to *identify what is occurring, research, identify biases*, use *logical reasoning, discern the relevance* of the information, and partake in an *unbiased discovery* by asking open-ended questions. Develop your own critical thinking process and begin to utilize it in *all* scenarios throughout your day. You will find that if you practice it enough, it will become second nature, and you will be able to better formulate unbiased conclusions by utilizing this process.

As an example of a scenario to critically think about, I was driving up the street on my way home and approached a red traffic light. I then came to a stop behind a sporty new Corvette. After admiring the car, I looked to my right and noticed a healthy-looking young woman, bound by a mask, in a car by herself. I began to think critically immediately. The identified issue was wearing a mask in a car by yourself. As a medical professional, I understand viruses are so tiny in comparison to the woven binding of face masks, and I asked myself the first critical thinking question. "Since viruses, being only nanometers in diameter, are too small to be stopped by a mask, how could it be logical to wear a mask to prevent inhaling any type of virus? I based this first question on substantiated research I already knew. Whom does this benefit? What could cause someone to do this? How could it prevent the exhalation from penetrating the surface based on the same logic? What other effects may it have? I continued using common sense as I thought critically. How could she be at risk if she was sitting alone and in her own space? What benefit could the mask be providing her in that setting? What is the most relevant information to substantiate this act? Isn't the body designed with the ability to fight off foreign objects, such as bacteria and viruses? As a matter of fact, isn't the body's own defense mechanism the *best* method of fighting them off? What would eventually be the effect on the body of blocking natural airflow into the lungs for an extended time? What would the inhaled mask fibers do to the body through time?[3] What are the masks made of?

My answer became very clear to me by using logical reasoning. I found no benefit to wearing a mask for a virus, especially in an environment of my own, by myself. It can be substantiated by performing research through trusted sources *with no agenda* other than to provide honest answers. What would cause this woman to be so fearful that she is wearing a mask, which is ineffective for viruses, and be afraid to breathe fresh air openly while riding solo in a confined vehicle, most likely being her own? *Fear* has been known to stand for *false events appearing real.* So why is she living in fear? Who instilled this fear in her? What is the source of the fear? What seems to be the reasoning for this fear? What appears to be the desired results of instilling fear in someone? Whom does this benefit? Do *they* have an agenda? Has the source of the fear overlooked, ignored, or left out information that doesn't support its agenda? Is the source using unnecessary language to cause fear? Is there a financial incentive for "the source"? An entirely new round of critical questions has evolved from the situation.

What causes people to become "sheeple" and blindly fall into a herd mentality without questioning the details behind it all? One method, as old as time yet obviously still effective, is intimidation by *fear.* If you scare people enough, you will be able to exert control over them, even to the point that they hide their faces while alone and seclude themselves from public interaction. That is a very severe depiction, yet a very real example, of what the world has recently experienced. Back in 2018 or 2019, would you ever have imagined willingly choosing to abandon all outside activity, including your commute to work, and "hiding" indoors from something that cannot even be seen? When you instill enough fear into people, they become willing to abandon critical thought and fall prey to the control of the ones leading the charge. How did the media participate in this event? Who funded the media? Is the media guilty of "outrage"?

Observe the volatile words they use to intimidate and manipulate you and play off of your emotions in an attempt to influence and control you. Words such as *outrage, corrupt, attacks,* and *urgent,* and phrases like *witch hunt, last chance,* and *breaking news* are all designed to appeal to your emotions and cause you to *submit* to their authority. They are meant to spark fear and cease your ability to think critically and use logic. Do you want to be constantly "riled up" by words such as these? How would your health be affected if you were constantly being inflamed? Why do they feel they have to strike you with emotional words to win your attention? *If "the source" believed in its own cause, there wouldn't be a need to use manipulation!* Do you feel the media's agenda is more important to them than *you* are as a person deserving of the truth and the ability to think for yourself and make your own sound decisions based on facts?

Ways to avoid getting caught up in the hysteria

1. *Become mindfully aware.* It all begins with awareness. Take a step back, or maybe two, and assess the situation. Be aware of the source of information. Who is causing the hysteria? What seems to be the reason for this happening? What seems to be the desired end result of the hysteria? How could this change things? Whom does this hysteria benefit? Does the source of this information appear to have an agenda? What is its agenda? Who is funding the source? Is the source overlooking, ignoring, or leaving out information that doesn't support its beliefs or claims? Is the source censoring people if they present with differing viewpoints? Is the source using persuasive or intimidating language to sway your perception? Are they relying on their ability to ignite your emotions for them to hook your attention and reel you into their side? Are they just trying to share unbiased and informative facts, or are they emotionally charged in their approach? What does it appear their goal is for you? To arouse your emotions? Ask yourself questions about the situation and make yourself aware of as much information as possible. Be open to all angles and possibilities. You may still agree to side with them after critically thinking, but at least allow yourself the opportunity to consider the occurrence from an unbiased perspective, asking questions in the process. Be aware of how they have chosen to engage with you. Why would someone be inclined to use emotion to win your support? Does this make you question the con-

tent, as well as the intent? Would the truth just speak for itself without emotion?

2. *Meditate.* Take time to regain control of your senses and emotions. Now that you are aware of what they are attempting to do, take some deep breaths and find a way to relax. There are many effective methods of meditation to choose from. Find a quiet and serene room to calm yourself and bring yourself to a peaceful high-frequency vibration. Clear your thoughts of all biases and prejudices and come to a place of honest contentment. Let your mind rest, and let your positive energy expand. Practice and explore various forms of meditation until you find the one that works best for you.

3. *Pray.* Just as you are able to clear your mind with meditation, you may clear your mind by focusing on your Creator and giving Him praise for all of your blessings. Place your trust in Him and the name of Jesus Christ. *"Let go and let God,"* as the saying goes. Be thankful for all that you have and are able to do. Praise and gratitude are two powerful qualities that have the ability to bring you to a place of tranquility in His precious name. Thank God for your freedom and ability to critically think without bias. Conversationally talk to God, and know He is with you at all times and through every event you encounter. Lean on Him and nail your fears and concerns to the cross of Jesus Christ. Allow the peace that is beyond all understanding to flow through every cell of your body. Pray for discernment as you wade through the ever-changing waters you encounter daily. Many wonderful prayers can be found online on every topic imaginable. Discover what prayers flow the best for you, or create your own. Let the Holy Spirit be your guide.

4. *Critically think.* Ask yourself questions regarding the situation, as discussed previously in this chapter. Who is doing what? What seems to be the reason for the situation happening? What are the desired end results for this hap-

pening? How could this change things? Whom does this benefit? Does the source of this information appear to have an agenda? What is the underlying agenda? Is the source overlooking, ignoring, or leaving out information that does not support its beliefs or claims? Is the source using unnecessary persuasive language to sway an audience's perception of the fact? Is it healthy for you to run from an "outraged" point of view? Does it benefit your family? Is it beneficial to your business or career? What might the consequences be if you submit to the intimidation of hysteria? What purpose would this serve? Do they care for your well-being? What causes people to use intimidation as a method of influence? Is it an ethical way to "try to get your way"? Is it professional? Are there any other ways to interpret the message? What are the details of the opposing view? Perform extensive research on this and on any other additional unbiased questions that come to mind. Analyze this information, verifying that the sources are valid and credible. Determine the relevance of the collected information and draw your own conclusions based on the unbiased raw data.

5. *Stop the flow of information.* Turn the television off. Close the news app, the Internet, or YouTube coverage. Is there another source of unbiased information you can choose? Perhaps you could back away from the information altogether? This is what I chose to do, and I went from being highly sensitized to being calm, relaxed, and peaceful, and I am engaging in a much more pleasurable way of life. Whenever I peek back in to see the "temperature" of the news sources, nothing has ever changed. Challenge yourself to shut off the valve on all news sources for a week. Assess the condition of your mind after this week. Assess your emotions. Do you notice any difference? Perhaps try it for two weeks—monitor, or even journal, regarding the results.

6. *Believe.* What is your belief system? Whom do you believe in? Is the method of hysteria aligned with your belief sys-

tem? Do you feel a sense of tranquility at the thought of pursuing the message? Your beliefs should lead you to a trusting place of serenity. Does this lead you there? Focus on your beliefs and let them direct your choices. Focus on what is good and what you know is right and true. Do not let others intimidate you or influence you under false pretenses. Know your core values, and let this be your guide. Define them and align with them. Put any questions you have through the critical thinking process.

7. *Distract.* What is important to you as a clinician? Is it more important to focus on your practice, the patients, and their specific needs? How about your family, loved ones, or even a hobby you enjoy? Is there a venue you could serve in to help others? There are many activities you could engage in that are more productive than allowing the hysteria to consume you. Pour your heart and soul into your family, business, career, church, or community service. Evaluate your priorities and disengage from the emotionally harmful noise of the media. Where can you be a blessing to others? Who can you positively impact? How can you leave an enlightened footprint in this world?

Misery loves company, and a potential goal of the news outlets is to combine and *conform* as many people as possible, as there is power in numbers. Once you add the factor of fear, you now have *control* as well. In that same mindset, isn't it time to band together (yet as individuals) with like-minded people in your own crusade, aligned with your values, and for the right reasons to protect your own freedoms and the patients and customers you serve? It is time to take action. Too much time has been spent in blind ignorance, closing eyes to the rapidly changing and progressing movement to erase history and live by fear and discontentedness, always looking for a reason to be highly sensitized. It's time to become fully aware of how your actions, choices, and decisions affect your patients or customers and what is being presented to them as well.

Critical thinking requires constantly updating your knowledge as you take in new information as it arises. You must look at your own biases and be logical in your reasoning. Look at things for yourself. Make your own decisions and be able to see more than one side of every issue. Think about what is happening around you, taking into consideration the allowance of false information (more about this will be addressed in the future chapter regarding propaganda) and whom this may benefit. Take the emotion away and think of the facts at hand.

If you listen to a major news outlet, are they known to be biased and one-sided? Does that logically sound reliable? Carefully listen to the input of others and consider it, yet know yourself enough to be able to make *your own* independent, informed, and logical decisions. As mentioned earlier, challenge yourself to debate each side separately to a winning position. Then, compare and evaluate your results. Be open-minded while using truth-seeking reasoning. There is an art to being able to disconfirm the claims of others, but it is done in such a way as to promote a common bond or shared fate. This will result in an *intensely* more powerful influence than intimidation or deceit. Use your mind without prejudice and fear, and learn to see things from opposing vantage points. Evaluate information from different perspectives, be open-minded for consideration, yet stand firm in your final, unprejudiced conclusions. Think for yourself, and *never* stop asking questions.

Responsibility to yourself means refusing to let others do your thinking, talking, and naming for you; it means learning to respect and use your own brains and instincts; hence, grappling with hard work.
—Adrienne Rich

The important thing is not to stop questioning. Curiosity has its own reason for existing.
—Albert Einstein

When we blindly adopt a religion, a political system, a literary dogma, we become automations. We cease to grow.

—Anais Nin

Critical thinking requires us to use our imagination, seeing things from perspectives other than our own and envisioning the likely consequences of our position.

—Bell Hooks

Nothing is more conducive to peace of mind than not having any opinions at all.

—Georg Christoph Lichtenberg

Whenever we hear an opinion and believe it, we make an agreement, and it becomes part of our belief system.

—Miguel Ruiz

People can be extremely intelligent, have taken a critical thinking course, and know logic inside and out. Yet they may just be clever debaters, not critical thinkers, because they are unwilling to look at their own biases.

—Carol Wade

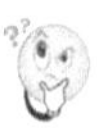

Reflect

1. What is critical thinking? What is the process of critical thinking?
2. Think about a medical topic that strikes an emotion. Now engage in critical thinking and ask yourself the series of critical thinking questions regarding that topic with an open mind and without prejudice. Now look at the situation from an opposing viewpoint.

3. What are the ways mentioned to avoid getting caught up in hysteria? What else can you add to this list?

4. How can you become more aware of potential manipulation in your environment, whether business or personal? How is your position affected by this manipulation? Are you able to remove your own bias and listen open-mindedly, considering opposing vantage points?

5. How do you use distractions to "break away" from emotionally charged information?

6. Find a meditation of choice and perform. Learn to transform your energy into positive, uplifting vibrations.

7. Practice asking critical questions in selected situations throughout each day.

CHAPTER 3

Where Does Your Obedience Lie?

*Control the manner in which a man interprets his world, and
you have gone a long way toward controlling his behavior.*
—Stanley Milgram

In 1961, psychologist Stanley Milgram began preparation for a series
of social psychology experiments, known as the Milgram experiments, measuring the willingness of men to obey an authority figure
who "*instructed them to perform acts conflicting with their personal
conscience.*"[4] The basis of these experiments was obedience to authority figures. The experiments began a year after the trial of Adolf
Eichmann in Jerusalem, with the intent of answering the questions,
"*Could it be that Eichmann and his million accomplices in the Holocaust
were just following orders? Could we call them all accomplices?*"
(Milgram 1974). Milgram was examining justifications for acts of
genocide offered by those accused at the World War II Nuremberg
War Criminal trials. The defense they used was based on the excuse
of "obedience." They claimed they were "just following orders" from
their superiors.

Participants in this experiment were led to believe they were
assisting an unrelated experiment, in which they had to administer
electric shocks, ranging from a mild initial shock of fifteen volts to
a four hundred fifty volts of a severe and dangerous shock to a person in another room who was a student learning. The shocks were

35

given upon each incorrect answer the student provided, with each one becoming progressively more intense. In reality, this other person was an actor. Yet the participant was led to believe that for each wrong answer, the student would receive an electrical shock at variably increasing volts, including a level considered fatal. In reality, no such punishment actually occurred. Prerecorded bloodcurdling sounds were prepared to add to the ambience of shock therapy.

It was found that a large percentage of participants would fully obey the instructions despite being uncomfortable. When the participant refused to administer a shock, the experimenter was to give a series of four orders to encourage and ensure that they continued. They displayed varying degrees of tension and stress as a result, including sweating, trembling, stuttering, biting their lips, groaning, nervous-laughing fits, seizures, and digging their fingernails. Every participant paused the experiment at least once to question it. After being assured by the experimenter, all participants continued with the experiment to three hundred volts, and two-thirds continued to the full four hundred fifty volts, which is at a potentially fatal level.

Milgram summarized the experiment in his 1974 article "The Perils of Obedience," writing,

> *The legal and philosophic aspects of obedience are of enormous importance, but they say very little about how most people behave in concrete situations. I set up a simple experiment at Yale University to test how much pain an ordinary citizen would inflict on another person simply because he was ordered to by an experimental scientist. Stark authority was pitted against the subjects' strongest moral imperatives against hurting others, and, with the subjects' ears ringing with the screams of the victims, authority won more often than not. The extreme willingness of adults to go to almost any lengths on the command of an authority constitutes the chief finding of the study and the fact most urgently demanding explanation. Ordinary people, simply doing their*

> *jobs, and without any particular hostility on their part, can become agents in a terrible destructive process. Moreover, even when the destructive effects of their work become patently clear, and they are asked to carry out actions incompatible with fundamental standards of morality, relatively few people have the resources needed to resist authority.*

Milgram was interested in finding out how far people would go in regard to obeying an instruction, even at the cost of harming another person. There came a point where the participants no longer saw themselves as responsible for their actions and proceeded to evoke what they thought was harmful onto another person. They became *a vessel* to carry out the instructions of another and submit to their authority, regardless of the consequence. Online research will lead you to many summaries of this experiment and related links for more information. Take some time to learn more about these experiments and the interpretations that resulted.

How do you see this happening in the world today? Can you see any examples in your life or the medical world, in general, that replicate, or are a variation of, these types of actions? What about regarding masking despite them being worthless to viruses? What is the reasoning behind this? What does science *really* say? Is this an example of blind obedience? What about "vaccinating" with a prototype experimental spike protein injection? Could this be blind obedience? Could it be that people will just blindly follow authority even at the risk of harming another person, including themselves? Are you able to set emotion aside and not become instantly biased and instead pursue research from opposing vantage points? What people in authority today have the opportunity to do this very same action? Have you ever been in this position, either as the one in authority or as the participant? How can you use critical thinking skills to reason out a logical answer to this dilemma?

Thoughts about the Milgram experiment

1. *Personalization.* The students were not "personalized" to the participants. There is a lot to be said about human nature and personal relationships. When you know someone intimately, the close bond creates an emotional attachment, making it more difficult to consider any sense of harm. Whereas in the experiments, not knowing the students personally allowed the participants to disconnect from the emotional aspect of the experiment, excluding the morality conscience variable that was present. This variable could be overcome in the name of science and via submission to the authority of the experimenter in charge. Do you think the results would have been different if there was a personal relationship between the participants and the students or, in this case, the actors? How would you have responded if you were a participant and you personally knew the student? What if the student was a family member or other loved one? What if you didn't know the student? What if *you were* the student? Would your relationship with the student bear any relevance on the decision you would make to, or not to, inflict harm on someone stemming from orders from an authority figure? What if this scenario involved a patient or customer? How about for a cause? How else might *you* be affected in your obedience to authority regarding issues of relationships with another? Would you dispense or administer a drug or vaccine without knowing what is actually in it or how it will affect a patient or customer you know well? How about someone you just met? How else might you be affected in your obedience to authority regarding issues of relationships with another? As the world becomes smaller and your freedoms continue to slip away, consider how you may be placed in a situation of obedience versus relationships. Perhaps if a similar occurrence happens in your work setting or in a group, social, or organizational setting, how would you respond? Consider how you would handle this

situation. What other critical thinking questions would you ask regarding the relationship factor?

2. *Obedience for a cause.* Most of the participants, even if reluctant, continued to inflict what they believed to be painful electric shocks upon students because that is what they were told to do. At one point or another, each one requested confirmation for assurance that they were doing the right thing and received it. Some were said to have proceeded in the name of science, believing they were responding to what they considered to be a "good cause." How would you react in this scenario? If presented with the same situation, would you blindly follow orders because you were told to do so, knowing you were severely hurting a random person? Or would you blindly follow orders in the name of science or for some other good cause? Would you critically think about whether or not it would be okay to inflict harm upon another innocent person for any reason? Would you obey like a loyal dog given an order? Or would your innate sense of morality prevent you from inflicting pain? Think of a scenario in your environment today where a cause of importance to you comes to mind. What are you willing to do for this cause? Would you dispense or administer a drug or vaccine without knowing its exact contents or harm it may incur for a cause? Would you allow harm to be inflicted upon someone else, whether known personally or not, for the sake of the cause? Whom would it benefit from this occurring? Would you have a moral dilemma if the reason was "for a cause"? What factors would make this okay in your mind? What factors would cause it not to be okay? How would you be affected if you were put in this situation? What if *you* were the one afflicted? How would you respond to the opposing side of the situation? Would your values come into play? How will you prepare for a similar situation that may potentially affect you today? What other critical thoughts come to mind?

3. *Herd mentality*. It has been said, and is proven to be true, that there is strength in numbers. As the participants observed their peers continuing to shock students despite the bloodcurdling pain responses, they claimed they felt more justified as they were following suit. In society today, do you see evidence of this type of behavior? When more and more people come together, is there a growing strength and conviction in their actions and inhibitions? As mentioned previously, people become "sheeple." Have you ever found yourself in a situation where you had a certain belief, but because of the crowd or group you were entangled with, you changed your choice and followed the crowd? What were the circumstances? How have you been influenced when the majority of people made it clear your choice or opinion was "wrong," and theirs was "right"? Did you stand your ground for what you believed in? It is difficult to go against the grain. Think about how determined salmon are to swim against the current to migrate back to their origins. They are not influenced by the current flowing in the opposite direction or by any other neighboring creatures among them. Nothing can prevent them from doing what they know they must do. What questions come to mind about how you react to differing crowds? What would happen if you stood your ground? Would you be willing to dispense or administer a harmful drug or unknown vaccine just because "everyone else is doing it"? Would you administer it to a pregnant woman, despite not having any clinical safety studies performed for subpopulations, including pregnant women or children? How far are you willing to go to find the facts? Would you be willing to harm another person based on the influence of a crowd or group? Or just because the media says it's okay and the entertainment community makes songs about its safety? Have you considered what their intentions are or what they are saying or thinking? Who funded them? Are you willing to administer an experimental vaccine with unknown con-

sequences and long-term adverse effects? Is there a "happy medium" between your viewpoint and theirs? Or deep down, do you still believe your original thought? How can you assess the situation and verify that you are aligning with your values? Your values are being challenged by an increasing rate (of alarm) daily. Identify your own moral code and belief system and align your thoughts and actions with your values. What do you need to do to intensify your convictions so you are less likely to sway from them? How can you remain strong in your own decisions based on your individual values? What other critical questions can you ask to explore this common scenario further?

4. *Intimidation.* There is a right and a wrong expression of authority. Recall your own innate sense of right and wrong—your code of morality. Your conscience will guide you if something is not right. It is important to have order in society and be obedient to the laws of the land. But how would you respond under intimidating circumstances? In the experiment, the participants were reassured that they were to follow the experimenter. He was in authority, and that in itself is indirectly an element of intimidation. What may have resulted if the rules weren't followed? Would there be a penalty? Would they become the student and be subjected to shocks? What part of intimidation is responsible for how someone reacts? In a similar scenario, how would you be affected with regard to intimidation? Would you react a certain way in anticipation of a negative result if you did not comply? What would happen if you obeyed, knowing there was an infliction of pain upon another person? What would happen to you if you disobeyed? Would you have a mental dilemma regarding your choices? How would the program be affected if you didn't obey? In society, are you strong enough to choose what you consider to be right despite a potentially intimidating outcome? How about despite intimidating pressure? Would you dispense or administer a harmful drug or *unknown* vaccine to a patient or customer based

on intimidation from someone in authority? What forms of intimidation reach and affect you? How do you respond to them? How can you overcome them? Think of a scenario today where you are being pressured in an intimidating manner. Are you being forced to take a drug or receive a vaccine against what you believe in? What are the circumstances? Was any important information regarding the product hidden from you or the public in general? What are your options in how to respond? Will your values be compromised? What are your values? Are they clearly defined? Are you willing to fight for them? Are you secure with who you are and willing to stand up for your values despite intimidation? If your values are not defined, how will you know what to stand up for? Prepare for how you would respond to intimidation in your current environment.

5. *Code of ethics.* Are you good with your word? Perhaps some of the participants continued because they committed themselves to the experiment. There was an ethical obligation to participate because they said they would. Do *you* do what you say and say what you do? What do you stand for? Whom do you stand for? What can you think of that would cause you to back out of what you said you would do? Where do you draw the line? What is your personal ethics code? How would you respond if you committed to something and then realized later that it violated your values somehow? What effects would this have on you? Where does your loyalty lie? How do your values affect the choices you make? Do you discover what a project or commitment entails before agreeing to pursue it? Do you research the effects of a drug or the ingredients of a vaccine and its adverse effects before choosing to dispense or administer it as per your oath to "first do no harm"? How can you prevent this situation from happening in the first place? What types of questions can you ask before you give your word or sign on the dotted line? Will you allow your values to be compromised?

6. *Location.* The setting may have been an influential factor in the experiment. Perhaps the industrial-like or professional lab-type setting had an effect on the participants. How would a formal location affect people? How might a "softer" setting make any difference? How would the technical equipment affect the participants? What effect would the sight and thought of the shock machine have on them? How about the proximity to the students? How are you affected by location? Do you respond differently in a "sterile" environment compared to a cozy, friendly environment? Would your values be defended differently in either case? What type of location would affect your decisions? Think about how you would respond to authority in your workplace versus in a family setting. Would you compromise your values in either one?

7. *Demeanor of the experimenter.* Perhaps the personality and demeanor of the one in charge swayed the degree of obedience. What effect could a certain personality have on the participants? What if the experimenter was gentle? What if the experimenter was brash and unapproachable? Would the personality have any effect at all? How do you handle situations when the one in authority has a distinct personality? How do you respond to gentle persuasion? How about a brazen persuasion? What would you do differently in each situation? Would you compromise the safety of your patient or customer? What if you discover the authority figure has a mentally challenged personality, such as narcissism? How would you respond knowing there is an embedded lack of concern or compassion for others? How is your performance affected by a shy leader? How about an aggressive leader? Have you ever let your values become compromised based on personality? How can you prepare yourself to do the "right" thing, in your eyes, no matter what personality you are dealing with?

8. *Settings.* Along with the location, perhaps the colors in the room affected the processing of information. Could the layout of the room and the chosen decor have affected the

"personality" of the room? How could the temperature affect the participants? Was the temperature warm, cool, or comfortable? What other sounds could be heard? Were there any defining scents or odors that could have affected the participants? How would the sound of the bloodcurdling screams affect them? How does a setting affect how you respond to authority? Would different settings change your responses in any way? How does temperature affect you? What if there were extreme temperatures? Would you be persuaded? How do lighting, colors, or smells affect your decision-making process? Would any of it have an effect on your obedience to authority? Would the running of only one specific news source in the setting persuade you to be obedient to their delivery of news or information? Would compassion prevail over obedience? Or would obedience stand as the decision made to honor authority despite setting variations? Is there a factor regarding the degree of the screams or moans? Would the intensity cause differing responses? What other factors could be influential to you? How can you prepare yourself to stand firm in your own values without prejudice or influence?

How far are you willing to go for the sake of obedience? Where does your obedience lie? Or maybe, *how* does your obedience *lie*? Do you have a clear delineation of what is acceptable and what borders on wrong or immoral? For the most part, it is important to be obedient to authority. However, when something occurs against your moral code, or you have this uneasy feeling or sense that something just isn't right, ask questions. Do you know what is in the products you are dispensing, administering, or prescribing? Have you spent time studying the research and clinical trials before administering the product to another human being? Do you know what the long-term side effects may be? Is the drug or vaccine "experimental"? Is propaganda required to be truthful? What research have you done to verify this? Are you following the crowd and assuming it's okay because others are dispensing the same drug?

Critically think about all aspects of the situation at hand and find as much information as possible. The patient or customer you serve deserves your full knowledge and responsibility for your part in their care. Consider both sides of the story and weigh the possibilities. Do not blindly follow the crowd if you do not know where they are going or if you know something isn't as it should be. Be authentic. Stand by your innate sense of right and wrong, and critically think your way to a resolution you can live with. Be brave and endure the process, guided wisely by *your* defined values.

> *The disappearance of a sense of responsibility is the most far-reaching consequence of submission to authority.*
> —Stanley Milgram

> *It may be that we are puppets—puppets controlled by the strings of society. But at least we are puppets with perception, with awareness. And perhaps our awareness is the first step to our liberation.*
> —Stanley Milgram

> *It is not so much the kind of person a man is as the kind of situation in which he finds himself that determines how he will act.*
> —Stanley Milgram

> *The essence in obedience consists in the fact that a person comes to view himself as an instrument for carrying out another person's wishes and he therefore no longer regards himself as responsible for his actions.*
> —Stanley Milgram

> *Each individual possesses a conscience which to a greater or lesser degree serves to restrain the unimpeded flow of impulse destructive to others. But when he merges his person into an organizational structure, a new creature replaces autonomous man, unhindered by the limitations of individual morality, freed of humane inhibition, mindful only of the sanctions of authority.*
> —Stanley Milgram

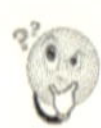

Reflect

1. What was the objective of the Milgram experiments?
2. Read three different versions of the experiments and the summaries they provide.
3. How do you respond to authority when it is aligned with your values?
4. How do you respond to authority when it is *not* aligned with your values?
5. Think about a controversial medical issue regarding obedience. Ask yourself three unbiased questions from the point of view that you favor. Next, ask yourself three unbiased questions from the opposing point of view, and consider all responses objectively and with an open mind.
6. How would you respond if you were in a group, and nine people thought one way, and you thought another? Would you alter your view, or would you stand your ground? What if they put pressure on you? What if only *you* put pressure on yourself because you thought differently? What critical thinking questions could you ask to assess the situation properly?
7. In a situation regarding obedience, how would you respond to volatile words like *outrage, shocking,* and *urgent*? Would you be intimidated to respond if someone was pressuring you? Ask yourself three critical thinking questions the next time you feel someone is trying to manipulate you by intimidation.
8. How can you stand by your innate sense of right and wrong and remain obedient? What if there was a time when what you considered "right" contradicted being "obedient"? What would you do?

CHAPTER 4

How Do You Decide?

You are an intelligent person with the ability to process large amounts of information. You have a tremendous capacity to think, analyze, and consider multiple and even complex situations and potential responses. Among other things, this separates you from other creatures, and each person has the opportunity to be authentic and think for himself or herself. So, how do you take advantage of this opportunity? What is your primary mode of decision-making? Do you have a hunger or drive for something? Or maybe it is based on a need or outside influence? Why might you be affected by the influence of others? Let's examine possible methods for decisions.

Methods of decision-making

1. *Critical thinking.* This is the desired method of decision-making. As mentioned earlier, critical thinking is a multifaceted method of asking unbiased questions from different angles of a situation. After you have clearly identified the situation or issue, gather facts and relevant information in an untainted manner and consider more than one vantage point. Without prejudice, seek to discover and collect content before formulating an educated inference. Be sure to collect as much information as possible and to ascertain the credibility of the sources you used for research

and the relevance of the contents. Understand the reasons you are drawn to one viewpoint versus another. Is there an influential reason? With critical thinking, you want to be a "blank slate" as you gather the data. Yet, as you have thoroughly processed all potential avenues, bring forth your innate sense of right and wrong as a guide, along with your carefully chosen objective evidence, in drawing a conclusion. Allow logic and common sense to be your GPS and navigate to an emotion-free decision in its origins.

2. *Intimidation.* Unfortunately, many things in life become, or perhaps always have been, intimidating. As you progress through different stages of life, the object of intimidation may change, yet there will likely be intimidating factors lurking. What comes to mind as an intimidating factor in your life? Or possibly, who? When you hear the word *intimidation*, what instinctively comes to mind? Is it a person, a financial event, a location, a status, or maybe a situational event? How do you handle intimidation? Do you give in to the influence and allow your values to be compromised? Or do you proceed with your own agenda despite it? Are some situations more intimidating than others? How do they affect you? Do you allow intimidation to control how you make decisions? How can you build up a tolerance against intimidation? How can you avoid intimidating people or circumstances? Prepare yourself to remain strong and convicted to your values, notwithstanding any attempts of intimidation from others. When possible, view things from both perspectives and consider all possibilities. Research for unbiased information, analyze all information you gather through trusted sources, and draw conclusions on the data at hand. Ultimately, critically think through intimidating factors, and do not allow them to compromise your values.

3. *Reputation.* Are you influenced by how people perceive you? This is very common in younger generations, as proven by social media, yet this can be influential to young

and old alike. It is human nature to want to be accepted by others. But is this a factor so powerful in your life that you will allow it to be the determining factor in making decisions? In particular, what if a morality issue was on the line? Would you base your decision on the issue by observing your conscience, or would you base it on how you will "look best" on social media? How much time do you spend on social media? Do you focus on the number of followers you have or how many people respond to "like" something you have posted? What causes the opinions of "social media" participants to value this digital form of acceptance more than in-person comradery? Do you partake for fun with no influential concern for responses, or do you rely on interactions for a form of popularity or acceptance? How about in a work setting? Do you make decisions a certain way because of your reputation? How about any other settings, such as a social or family situation? Does your reputation in any setting affect how you make decisions? Do you, or are you willing to, compromise your values for your reputation?

4. *Herd mentality.* There truly is power in numbers, and inhibitions can be altered as well. For whatever reason, some people feel "safe" when they are within a group and may be inclined to "become" what they are all about. A good example of this is found in gangs. The premise of a gang is to find security in a group of people and feel accepted. In the process, the group generally thinks as one unit—*group think*—in the hopes and expectation of acceptance. Often, they may not even be *permitted* to think for themselves. They lost their individuality and gave in to conformity. Possibly, at this point, there may even be a *penalty* if they attempt to leave the group. There are many other groups of like-minded people as well. In a group, it is important to have the freedom and safety to be still able to think and speak for yourself. Are you permitted to be authentic? Do you follow in line with the majority? Who benefits from

being in the group? Who controls the group? What are your reasons for being in the group? Do you consider all information and then formulate your own opinion? If the majority is in agreement, which violates your morals, how do you respond? If you respond with an opposing view, how do they respond to you? Would you still be accepted? Or would you be in danger? Is the group mellow or volatile? What seems to be the agenda of the group? Are you strong enough to stand up for your own beliefs and make independent decisions?

5. *Peer pressure.* Peer pressure is not just a concern in the school system for preteens or teenagers. It also exists in every age group and in every realm. The premise of peer pressure, like herd mentality, is also to be accepted by others. Sometimes you may be challenged to do something or act in a certain way based on the promptings of someone else. Perhaps it is a coworker or even a boss. It could stem from a group of friends or even family. Whatever the source, how are you affected by pressure from peers? Who is applying the pressure? What seems to be the desired goal of the pressure? How does the pressure affect your ability to make decisions? Do you allow them to influence you and sway your decisions? Do you consider the validity of their request or insistence? Identify the situation and allow yourself to listen to their side of the issue. Consider the source, and if more information is needed to substantiate the claim, proceed in performing your own individual research. Find out as many facts regarding the situation as possible. Evaluate all of the data. Next, align the information with your values. What are potential options to resolve the situation? Independently draw your own conclusions. Did you come to the same conclusions as they did using an unbiased, critical thinking method? If your conclusions differ, are you confident enough to stand firm in your decision that aligns with your values? What types of pressures from other people affect you? What are some ways you can

avoid peer pressure in the first place? How can you create an environment where peer pressure is minimized, if not eliminated altogether?

6. *Financial advantage.* Financial incentives are intriguing and most likely appealing. But what is the premise of the incentive? Is it in exchange for a worthy service, object, or event? Or is there a persuasive nature, requesting you to sway to a certain side of an issue? How might you be influenced by a financial persuasion, even if it is set against your sense of what is right? Or are you able to choose the "right" option, despite a prosperous reward for choosing the "wrong" side? Is there a dollar amount that is a deciding factor? Are there any other extenuating circumstances that would cause you to tag on a decision based on a financial advantage? How would you handle a significantly prosperous request that clashed with your morals? How can you guard yourself against allowing a financial incentive to sway your decisions when your values are concerned?

7. *Fear.* Fear encompasses numerous possibilities, each different for every individual. What are some of your fears? What is your biggest fear? Do you have a fear of abandonment or of being alone? Do you have a fear of missing out on something (FoMo)? Or maybe you have a fear of reprisal if you do not blindly follow a boss's or hospital system's orders? Sometimes a fear may develop with the knowledge you obtain about others. Personally, I worked for a person whom I later found out had a criminal background in both assaults and possessing illegally obtained narcotics. While it is questionable how she ever obtained a leadership role in an addiction clinic in the first place, this led her to "lead" based on her own fear of inadequacy. Once I pieced this all together, including the knowledge of an additional peer who had a history of a felony charge for drug addiction and theft, in this same addiction clinic and who therefore operated out of fear of losing her own position and not obtaining another one, I chose to remove myself from

this situation. Sometimes the fear lies in the other party, and you must protect your own safety, good name, and livelihood. Or maybe there is a general fear, such as a fear of the unknown. There may be a fear derived from not being accepted or perhaps a fear of harm if you don't conform to a certain way or opinion. Perhaps it's just a fear of being wrong. Identify your greatest fear. How would this fear shape the way you make decisions if it came into play? Would it cause you to make a decision differently than if the fear were not present? Would it cause you to make a decision against your morals or belief system? Would any of your values be compromised? How can you *reframe* this fear and see it in a new light? Is there any conditioning you can perform or things to avoid to desensitize, or even remove, yourself from the fear? Identify ways to separate this fear from your decision-making opportunities.

8. *Emotionally charged.* An emotionally charged person, especially a group, could distinctly impact a situation. People who are emotionally charged often respond *based* on emotions rather than logic. It is difficult not to be affected by this type of volatile demeanor, especially if you are a well-controlled person. The negative vibrations are infectious, and they spread rapidly. Many movements today are actually *based* on emotions themselves rather than on logic. How do you respond when you are with someone running on high emotions? Are you influenced to side with them just to keep the peace? Or maybe out of fear? How do you respond when you are within a group that becomes highly charged? Would you tend to conform to the intense energy? Are you still able to hold true to your beliefs? How would you handle the emotional intensity if it was in contrast to your values? Identify ways you could remove yourself from the emotion in this type of situation and allow yourself to critically think your way to an unbiased resolution.

9. *Spiritually charged.* Sometimes there is a spiritual realm that may draw people to a decision. It may not necessarily be

based on what is right versus wrong, but rather, it is *spiritually* driven. This method may be built on passion or a desire, as well as with an emotional attachment. How would you handle something of this persuasion? Do you still respond based on your core values? Perhaps it's a matter of *how* you respond that is of concern. Have you ever been overly passionate about a cause you believe in and responded in a way you normally wouldn't have? Do you let passion alter the way you respond? How might you respond if your beliefs were being jeopardized? Are you able to look at both sides indiscriminately? What information can you gather that might help you reach a logical conclusion? How can you hold your own emotions at bay while taking an unbiased look at both sides? How can you avoid potential situations that contradict your values in the first place? Collect as much information as possible without prejudice, then draw a logical solution rather than "drinking the Kool-Aid."

10. *Loyalty.* Loyalty is an admirable character quality to possess if it is aligned with your values. What or who are you loyal to? What are the reasons for the loyalty? To what extent will you devote your allegiance? What would you do if the object of your loyalty was compromised? How would you respond if your loyalty were challenged? Would your loyalty trump your values? What is the opposing perspective on the situation? Is there a reasonable premise? Will this cause you to alter how you respond? How far would you take loyalty when it coincides with your values? How far would you take it if it *contradicted* your values? If trust were broken, how would you handle the situation? Will your loyalty ever cause you to compromise your values? How does loyalty affect how you make decisions?

11. *Obedience.* Stanley Milgram based his experiments on the effects of human nature on obedience. How do you relate to the participants in Milgram's experiments? Would obedience to an authority figure affect your decision to do something against your values? What about obedience

to someone you trust and love? Could that possibly lead you to compromise your values? Is there a scenario that would cause you to alter your belief system in the name of obedience? Are you obedient without question? Or do you critically think about including your values in making a decision? Where and to what extent does your obedience lie? Gather as much information as necessary to provide the proper knowledge for making your decision. In society, elites take more power upon themselves than "We the People" ever gave them. Be prepared to perform detailed research before ever blindly obeying an authority that lies opposite your values. How can you prepare for times like this? How does obedience affect your decision-making process?

12. *Need- or desire-based.* Do you allow a need or desire to compromise your decisions? Will you go against your beliefs to satisfy a need? What about a desire? Are you willing to alter a decision and go against your values to attain an object in need or one you "want"? Be aware that there may be others around you who are capable of compromising what is right, such as mentioned in the "fear" scenario previously. Perhaps someone you work with operates on a "need" to protect their own positions, thereby compromising their values. Do you allow others who have compromised their values to affect your decisions? Perhaps there are some you would and some you would not. How would you handle these types of situations? What are some of your strong needs or desires? How do you evaluate their importance compared to your values? Do you take your values into consideration and make a logical decision? Do you have control over your wants and needs? If not, what can you do to gain control over them? How will you compare opposing sides and evaluate these situations in an unbiased manner? How do your needs and desires affect your decision-making process?

13. *Insecurity.* Many forms of insecurities have the potential to influence decisions. Insecurity, in general, can lead people to act in peculiar ways. Perhaps you want to be liked or accepted, or do *not* want to stand out in a crowd, or *do* want to stand out as unique. Perhaps it is based on talent or the work that you do. Have you ever let insecurity sway a decision that you made? What was the premise of the insecurity? Who was involved? Who benefited from this decision? Is there a certain insecurity that would cause you to set aside your values? What would you do if the insecurity presented itself even though you would not be harmed by choosing your values? Are you stronger than your insecurity? How do insecure people affect you? Are you still able to make decisions aligned with your values while around them? How can you find out more information regarding the opposing sides of insecurity? Collect as much information as possible, and then evaluate the data. How can you work toward resolving the insecurity so it is no longer an issue? How can you prepare so insecurity is not an issue when making decisions?

There are many different factors behind the process of making a decision. Perhaps you have encountered half, or even all, of the mentioned conditions at some point in your life. No matter what you are experiencing or how you approach the decision, employ critical thinking methods before you make your ultimate decisions. Who is doing what? What seems to be the reason for this happening? What are the potential or desired end results? How could they possibly change? Whom does this benefit? Does the source of this information appear to have an agenda? What is the agenda? Is the source overlooking, ignoring, or leaving out information that doesn't support its beliefs or claims? Is the source using unnecessary language to sway an audience's perception of a fact? How are your values affected? What would it look like through the eyes of the opposing side? How can you meet them in the middle with a compromise without bending your values? What are other potential responses?

Is there anything clouding your judgment? Do you see the situation through unbiased eyes? Are you allowing other people or things to affect your decision? Are you using logic? Utilizing credible and reliable resources, research and gather as much relevant information as possible. Analyze and extrapolate your own conclusions based on the raw data.

> *We all make choices, but in the end, our choices make us.*
> —Ken Levine

> *We are free to choose our paths, but we can't choose*
> *the consequences that come with them.*
> —Sean Covey

> *Good and evil both increase at compound interest. That is why the little*
> *decisions you and I make every day are of such infinite importance.*
> —C. S. Lewis

> *If, before every action, we were to begin by weighing up*
> *the consequences, thinking about them in earnest, first the*
> *immediate consequences, then the probable, then the possible,*
> *then the imaginable ones, we should never move beyond*
> *the point where our first thought brought us to a halt.*
> —José Saramago

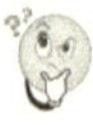

Reflect

1. What is your primary mode of decision-making? Name factors that could affect how you make your decisions.
2. Name someone you know who practices critical thinking in his or her decision-making opportunities. How does this process affect their decision outcomes?

3. How can you incorporate more critical thinking and less influential distractions into your decisions?
4. Think of a time when you allowed intimidation to affect your decision-making. How can you reframe this by critically thinking?
5. How about reputation? Herd mentality? Peer pressure? Financial advantage? Fear? Emotionally charged? Spiritually charged? Loyalty? Obedience? Need- or desire-based? Insecurity? How can you reframe each of these methods by critically thinking?

CHAPTER 5

What Happened in
Nineteen Eighty-Four?

We are coming to a time in the creation of our own "history" where there is a decision to be made between individuality and conformity. There is a battle between personal freedom and political repression. Faced with biased media outlets and additional forms of psychological intimidation, individual freedoms are becoming increasingly "challenged." George Orwell had an astounding "intuition," or perhaps a "premonition," as he wrote the infamous book *Nineteen Eighty-Four* in 1949.

Orwell's novel explored themes such as totalitarianism, communism, and a *dystopian* future. *"A dystopia refers to a fictional place that is characterized by the universally miserable conditions under which its citizens live, usually under the guise of utopia."*[5] In Orwell's setting, the creation of this particular fictional dystopia was both from war and government, with the main "superstate," *Oceania*, in a constant state of war. The fictional dictator of *Oceania* is Big Brother, which is symbolic and designed to terrify the population into submission by those in power. This is the premise of the famous saying, "Big Brother is watching you," which is in reference to the constant surveillance of the people.

The basis of the story revolves around the main character, Winston Smith, and his journey and struggle to gain individual freedom, which essentially never did happen. The novel also included a new language created by the government, *Newspeak*, intending to *suppress free thought*. Orwell realized the systems of communism and socialism would have difficulty succeeding when put into practice because the people in authority were generally greedy and *obsessed* with power and control. Orwell also wrote *Animal Farm* (1945), and along with *Nineteen Eighty-Four*, both novels blasted the totalitarian regimes and the control they seek over their citizens to basically turn them into submissive herds of sheep, or as some would say, "sheeple."

The novel continued with the mission to bring about change for the people who resembled Soviet Union communism and to *purge history* from the minds of the citizens. There are many more details and aspects of both *Nineteen Eight-Four* and *Animal Farm* that I encourage you to study for yourself. Take some time to read or listen to both of these novels written by George Orwell. Also, read numerous summaries and interpretations of each, and compare and contrast these novels to the circumstances of our culture, society, and government today. Critically think about all aspects mentioned, including dystopia, submission by fear, constant surveillance, suppression of speech and free thought, obsession with power and control, and purging history, so you are able to make logical and informed decisions to the best of your ability.

Who is doing what in the novels? Who is doing what in society? What seems to be the reason for this happening in the novels? What about in society? What are the end results of the novels? What are the desired or implied end results in society? How could these results change in either case? Does any of this concern you?

Your own independent research is key when comparing arguments, according to Will Erstad.[6] How will you independently verify the context or content? What sources will you use? How will you evaluate them? Develop an eye for "unsourced claims" so you can easily sort them out. Not all sources are equally valid; learn the differences between them. Evaluate the information *objectively*, and be sure to evaluate *both* sides of the argument. Set aside your own bias so your judgment is not clouded. Identify the evidence that forms your beliefs, if possible.

Are your sources credible? In the evaluation of the information, who does the content benefit? Does the source appear to have an agenda? Does there appear to be any information excluded or overlooked? Is there bias or persuasion in the language? Assess the information and draw your conclusion based on the data. Extrapolate and discover potential outcomes, understanding that your inference will be made on the information collected and that additional information may lead to different conclusions. The more information gathered, the easier it will be to formulate an educated conclusion.

What information is most relevant to your research? How will you determine relevance? What information are you seeking to discover? What is your end goal? These are all very important questions to ask as you collect raw data in your desire to come to your own educated and individually thought-out conclusion. Learn to think critically in all matters of importance. Draw your own conclusions and question the intent and content of others. Know your own reasonings and intentions and seek to become fluent in critical thinking.

What are your thoughts about individuality versus conformity? What is the meaning of each of these words? Describe the way of life involved under each of these headings. Create different scenarios and consider each label throughout each scenario. Who benefits from individuality? Who benefits from conformity? Picture yourself in a setting where everyone is their own person, choosing their own career, hobbies, activities, foods, and friends. Now, visualize a setting where everyone is dressed the same, performing the same job, participating in the same hobby and activities, eating the same food, and interacting with the same people, all presented to you without your selection. How would you feel about your ability to choose versus being presented with things *without* your choice? How would you benefit in either situation? How might you begin to lose yourself when your ability to choose is taken away? What is your ideal situation?

Have you ever wondered, especially recently, what it would be like to have free thought suppressed? How about free speech in the form of censorship simply because you may not think the way someone else wants or expects you to? It's one thing if you are on the side of the one doing the suppressing, but what if you are the one being suppressed? Does this go against the freedom promised to you in the US Constitution? Does it ever appear that the news outlets treat you like part of the "herd," treating you like a sheep and expecting conformity and submission?

Allow yourself to continue to create a few more scenarios, comparing and contrasting the differences between individuality and conformity. What are your thoughts about being part of a herd mentality? What are your thoughts about freedom? Be objective as you carefully consider each side. What research can you perform to learn more about the differences between the two? How do each of these stories bring light to the issue of individuality versus conformity? In the stories, what do you think about the erasing of history from their minds? What do you think about the plan to erase history from your mind? What do you think about your history being erased from the minds of the following generation? Where do your thoughts lead you regarding this exercise? Continue to observe the scenarios without prejudice by critically thinking about them and presenting yourself with lots of questions and extensive research. Draw your own conclusions after evaluating all of your research.

Every record has been destroyed or falsified, every book rewritten,
every picture has been repainted, every statue and street building
has been renamed, every date has been altered. And the process is
continuing day by day and minute by minute. History has stopped.
Nothing exists except an endless present in which Party is always right.
—George Orwell

Until they become conscious, they will never rebel, and until
after they have rebelled, they cannot become conscious.
—George Orwell

Perhaps one did not want to be loved so much as to be understood.
—George Orwell

Now I will tell you the answer to my question. It is this. The Party seeks power entirely for its own sake. We are not interested in the good of others; we are interested solely in power, pure power. What pure power means you will understand presently. We are different from the oligarchies of the past in that we know what we are doing. All the others, even those who resembled ourselves, were cowards and hypocrites. The German Nazis and the Russian Communists came very close to us in their methods, but they never had the courage to recognize their own motives. They pretended, perhaps they even believed, that they had seized power unwillingly and for a limited time, and that just around the corner there lay a paradise where human beings would be free and equal. We are not like that. We know that no one ever seizes power with the intention of relinquishing it. Power is not a means; it's an end. One does not establish a dictatorship in order to safeguard a revolution; one makes the revolution in order to establish the dictatorship. The object of persecution is persecution. The object of torture is torture. The object of power is power. Now you begin to understand me.

—George Orwell

Being in a minority, even a minority of one, did not make you mad. There was truth and there was untruth, and if you clung to the truth even against the whole world, you were not mad.

—George Orwell

Big Brother is Watching You.

—George Orwell

Nothing was your own except the few cubic centimeters inside your mind.

—George Orwell

It was possible, no doubt, to imagine a society in which wealth, in the sense of personal possessions and luxuries, should be evenly distributed, while power remained in the hands of a small privileged caste. But in practice such a society could not long remain stable. For if leisure and security were enjoyed by all alike, the great mass of human beings who are normally stupefied by poverty would become literate and would learn to think for themselves; and when once they had done this, they would sooner or later realize that the privileged minority had no function, and they would sweep it away. In the long run, a hierarchical society was only possible on a basis of poverty and ignorance.

—George Orwell

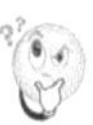

Reflect

1. Read *Nineteen Eighty-Four* and *Animal Farm* by George Orwell. Summarize the key elements of each story. What thoughts come to mind from each of them?

2. How does each story compare and contrast to the culture you live in today? Knowing the books were written in 1949 and 1945, respectively, what are your thoughts regarding George Orwell's "premonition" of the direction society could take?

3. What sources did you use to evaluate? What information do you see as most relevant? How does this affect you?

4. What is your biggest concern regarding the conclusions you came to? What is the premise of your concern? How might this affect your practice?

5. How will you use this information in your daily life? Does it change how you perceive things? Is there anything that surprises you?

CHAPTER 6

Why All the Propaganda?

What is the purpose of propaganda, and where did it all begin? Propaganda has become a powerful tool used to gain approval. It is a way to sway the masses through all available media sources by those in a position to do so, including the military! While the origin, or its inception, was innocent enough back in 1622, according to Edward Bernays in his book *Propaganda*, it has now evolved into an entity of "troubling connotation," as it has become a method of *manipulation* and intended enterprise.[7] Propaganda is used today as a method of *controlling* how *you* think and act.

In 2013, the president of the United States signed the Smith-Mundt Modernization Act of 2012 into law, which was part of the 2013 National Defense Authorization Act, which essentially *legalized lying* to the public for propaganda purposes![8] "*Today, the military is more focused on manipulating news and commentary on the internet, especially social media, by posting material and images without necessarily claiming ownership.*" News and journalist reporting are now *no longer required* to be factual! This is all befitting of George Orwell's literary work discussed in the previous chapter, known as *Nineteen Eighty-Four*. The US government is now propagandizing the American people in many ways, including through the control of major media outlets, Big Pharma, social media, and the Tech Giants. Take some time to read *Propaganda, Nineteen Eighty-Four, Animal Farm, United States of Fear*, the Smith-Mundt Modernization Act,

Turtles All the Way Down,[9] and many other such sources of your own choosing.

While you may have already noticed that the media is not relaying factual content, were you aware that they have been given *permission* and have even been encouraged to *deliberately deceive* you? Apply critical thinking methods to this topic. Why did this happen? Who is involved in the deception? What is the agenda behind the deception? Who will benefit from the deception? What are the underlying reasons for the deception? Why would a law be passed to allow government and communication sources to lie to the American people? Why would it be okay for the media to lie to the American people? What would their perspective potentially be regarding this topic? Do they have *your* best interests in mind? How about your patients? What is your perspective on this topic? What is *your* response to the permission to deceive to persuade you? How does this affect you? How is this going to reconfigure your thoughts as you listen to the media outlets from now on? Will you apply critical thinking questions to each piece of media you encounter from this point forward? What current practices will you change in response to this knowledge? How are you affected by manipulative information? How have they been effective in convincing you to believe in their content? What methods do you apply to verify the legitimacy of the content? How do you know the truth behind the content? Will you think differently regarding their information? How can you better prepare to handle more and more media outlets as they conform to the freedom to deceive? Knowing their intent is to *control* you, how will you respond? Will you allow them to control you and connect the dots for you? Or will you take steps of awareness and program your mind to automatically *question the intent* of the content?

It is important to arm yourself with the necessary information based on your decision. What research will you do to verify sources and content? Be careful and methodical as you analyze your research. It is helpful first to understand how manipulation is used.

Keys to successful manipulation

1. *Utilizing and controlling appropriate media outlets.* The government and other political venues have successfully gained control of nearly all major news and media outlets. This is not an accidental occurrence. And it is also not a sudden occurrence. When did you come to an awareness that this is happening? Who owns the different outlets? Take some time and research for yourself. What are the connections among the owners? What is the agenda of having a monopoly over major media sources? What are the possible outcomes of the monopoly? How could, or does, this affect you? What conclusion do you come to regarding this movement of control? What are the possible benefits of total control? What are the disadvantages of total control? Whom are they trying to manipulate? What seems to be the reason for the manipulation? What are the desired end results of doing this? How could this change things? How does *any* monopoly have positive outcomes? Whom does the manipulation benefit? Does the source of the media outlets appear to have an agenda regarding the manipulation? Are they overlooking, ignoring, or leaving out information that doesn't support their agenda? Are they censoring anyone who presents with an opposing viewpoint? Are they using unnecessary persuasive language to sway the audience's perception of a fact? How will you research the content provided? How will you verify the validity of the information? Ensure you seek the most relevant information as you collect as much data as possible. Evaluate all of the raw data and extrapolate potential outcomes. Draw your own conclusions. Do you realize you are not as "free" as you once thought you were?

2. *Taking away the individual.* The government is trying desperately and is succeeding in manipulating people into forming groups and having a group mentality. They are *afraid* to have people think and act individually and be a

strong force of their own with their own thoughts, agenda, and individual actions. People can be very powerful when they use their own logic and intellect—so powerful, in fact, that they are feared. Thus, movements have been well underway to promote groups of people, encouraging them to pick an "identity" or in some way be a part of a group and engage in emotional bonds to keep their focus on that group rather than realizing that *individual* rights are being absorbed by the government, thereby *weakening* the people as a whole. *They* are *dividing* us. Being a part of a group is not a concern until it becomes focused on an *emotional* endeavor, giving more and more power to the *governing body* rather than to the rights of the *individual*. It is all a *loss of control* for the people and *more strength* for the government. Who is in charge of promoting groupthink? What seems to be the reason for this happening? What appears to be the desired end results of groupthink? How could this change things? Whom does this benefit? Does the source of this information appear to have an underlying agenda? Is the agenda to help, nourish, encourage, and grow you? Or is the agenda meant to divide people against one another? Is the source overlooking, ignoring, or leaving out information that doesn't support its agenda? Is the source using unnecessary persuasive language to sway your perception of a fact? What research can be performed from a neutral and unbiased source to find out more information? What would the result be of weakening the unity of the people as a whole? How can we all still be our own individuals yet stand *together* as *individuals, strengthening one another* as a country rather than *handing over control* to the government? What would the benefits be if we could all be ourselves as individuals and support one another and not give over our control to the government? What if we relinquished "group thinking" and used our *individual* power and ability to critically think and analyze situations with the goal of a *stronger and unified* country?

3. *Developing fear in people.* Fear is the *primary* way to gain *control over* people. When people *feel* afraid or in some way harmed, they quickly bow down to authority. Look how easy it is to create a worldwide stir and make people "want" to stay home and wear masks even while alone in a desolate place, such as their own vehicle. Fear is the primary way to create a movement on such a large scale. Can you think of any way to make people willingly concede to having spiked protein factories injected into them, in some cases two, three, four, and even five times? What research has been done to learn more about the source of the virus? How about the experimental spiked protein "vaccine"? Have you found evidence proving the virus has actually been around for quite a while *prior* to the claim? What news outlet did you gather information about it from upon discovering it? Was the information you collected from a "major news outlet," which now, as you know, has permission and encouragement to *deceive*? How effective were the volatile words (*urgent, critical, deadly, pandemic*) at achieving the desired effect—gaining *control* over people? Who is stirring up fear? How effective is fear in forcing people to do something? What seems to be the underlying reason for this happening? What appears to be the desired end result of the fear? How could this change things? Whom does the fear benefit? Is there some sort of funding involved or a financial incentive? Does the source of this information appear to have an agenda? Is the source overlooking, ignoring, or leaving out information that doesn't support its agenda? Is the source censoring anyone who presents with a differing viewpoint? Is the source using unnecessary and persuasive language to sway the audience's perception of the facts? Was the media "fair and unbiased"? Where can you go to find scientific evidence? What information can morticians, embalmers, and funeral directors provide who have seen the *resulting evidence* of the claims and, in this case, the *experimental* vaccine?[10] How can you undergo

unbiased research and find answers for yourself? Search for as many resources as possible from both sides of the argument. Be sure to find credible sources to discover the most relevant information regarding this data and gather as much information as possible. Use your ability to infer and draw conclusions after evaluating all of the data.

4. *Create a solution.* Once fear is instilled, the next step is to create a solution. For instance, as popular computer software became available decades ago, computers and systems ran amazingly well. Perhaps too well. How can this continue to be profitable? What could make it *more* profitable? How about a virus, so now more products could be created and purchased to resolve the new issue? Thus, the invention of computer viruses and another lucrative endeavor. How about for a human-infected virus? What if a virus was used as a bioweapon, or at least "*in theory*"? Then, there would be a demand for a "vaccine" to counter the virus. Governing bodies have chosen this same method of creating a problem and then creating a solution for generations. As it stands, it is extremely desirable to get any vaccine approved for the childhood list of vaccines. This is a goal of Big Pharma to secure *enormous* profits.[11] It then becomes a money factory. Who is creating a solution? Who is funding the research to make this possible? What seems to be the claim for the solution? What are the desired end results of the solution? How could this change things? Whom does the solution benefit? Is there extensive research proving the safety of the solution? Where can you find credible data regarding the safety of the solution? Does the source of the solution appear to have an agenda? Is there a monetary benefit to the source of the solution? Are there alternate solutions? Who else may benefit? Is there a secondary agenda? Is the source overlooking, ignoring, falsifying, or leaving out information that does not support its claim? Is there censorship for anyone with opposing views? Is the source of the solution using persuasive language to sway people's

perception of the facts? What research can you perform using valid, detailed, and unbiased sources? Where can you find reliable and the most relevant information? Always, *always* perform your own research, and choose credible and multiple sources. Evaluate all of the information collected and draw your own conclusions.

5. *Changing or creating laws to fit the agenda.* Just as occurred in 2013, a method of manipulation may be established by changing laws to fit an agenda. This could happen at any level, but people already in authority generally have the power to do this. Sure enough, in 2013, the Act was signed to *allow and encourage* the media to deceive the American people through propaganda. When you can force people to be subjected to certain things, there is a greater chance that submission to the influence will occur. What situation can you think of in which a law or rule was established or adjusted to fit someone else's specific agenda? Who changed the laws? What seems to be the reason for the changes? What are the desired end results of changing the law? How could this change things? Who received benefits from this occurrence? How are you affected by it? Does the source of the changed laws appear to have an agenda? What does it appear to be? Is the source stacking hidden clauses buried deep within another law to ensure its passage? Is the source overlooking, ignoring, or leaving out pertinent information that does not support its claim? Is there censoring if someone presents with an opposing vantage point? Is the source using unnecessarily persuasive language to sway the people's perception of facts? How can you evaluate the situation so you understand the terms? What do you see if you look at things from the opposing perspective? How can you protect yourself from manipulation? How do you know when you are being controlled, deceived, or manipulated? Where can you find unbiased information? Gather as much data as possible from credible sources. Use your ability to infer to discover potential conclusions.

6. *Taking control of positions of power.* To influence a massive number of people, it is necessary to be in a position of power or know someone in such a position. How can a position of power give an extra advantage? Who is the main target of interest for this position? What is the particular position? What seems to be the reason for the certain position? Is it a position of power? Who funded the campaign? What connection or involvement do they have? What or who does the position control? What appears to be the desired end result of being in the position? How could this change things? Will they be working in your favor? Who else might they be working for? What does the position have authority over? Are the policies or rules created and enforced for the best interest of the people being served? Who benefits from them being in this position? Who benefits from their decisions? How does this affect you? What appears to be the agenda of being in this position? Do there appear to be any hidden agendas? How does "the source" benefit from being in this position? How can you find out the intent of the actions? Are there alternate people interested in this position? Who is the best qualified for this position? Does the source resort to downplaying or humiliating its opponent to make itself look better for the position? Is there any effort for deception in attaining this position? Does the source use persuasive language to sway the people's perception of the facts? What is the basis for their campaign or selection? Is there censorship involved to help attain the position? Do extensive research for every elected official promoting something questionable. Find sources of information regarding all people running for a position of power, including opposing sides. Put aside your biases and prejudices, and gather information from multiple, credible, and varying resources. Collect as much information as possible. Determine which information is most relevant, evaluate and analyze all data, extrapolate and dis-

cover facts, and then draw your own conclusions without prejudice or influence from anyone else.

7. *Developing a dependency within people.* Submission can be gained by developing a dependency within the people toward those in authority. This can be developed through numerous avenues, including fear, group thinking, and deceit from the media. Successful leadership involves the one in the position of authority *serving* the needs of those who did the electing. Unfortunately, governing officials have somehow abused their power and turned the positions into *self-serving agendas* that involve manipulating the people to serve *their* needs and desires. Who is working for whom? Who is causing a dependency? Why might there be a need for dependency? What seems to be the desired end result of the dependency? How could this change things? Who is the focus of the agenda? How can you become more independent? How does the government use the media to create dependency within people? Who benefits from this dependency? How does this affect you? What happens if the majority of people become dependent on the government? Will this affect your freedom? How can you find relevant and unbiased information about this topic? Collect as much information as possible regarding dependency. Evaluate and analyze the information. Draw your own conclusions using your own unbiased logic.

8. *Creating controversy.* Did you happen to notice that the real *enhanced* issue of racism, fascism, and other politically overutilized *isms* only occurred when the first black president came into office and *promoted and exploited* this idea? Do not take my word for it, but instead, do your own research and gather facts regarding this topic. If you divide the country and the people, the government becomes *stronger*, and the people become *weaker*. So many groups have fallen for this tactic and played right into the hands of the instigators. There is now more reliance *by* the people *on* the government. This is *exactly* the intent of the effort. In this

sense, the government is becoming *more* powerful. Who started the instigating? What might the motives be for this movement of creating *emotional-based* controversies? Who benefits from a stronger government and weaker people? What is the desired outcome of controversy among the people? How does the government become stronger as the people become weaker? What are the potential outcomes of this result? How does this concern you? How do you fit into this scenario? What research can you do to find out facts for clarification? What sources can you identify that will provide unbiased information? What would happen if the government and media stopped promoting the idea of these *isms*? Collect as much data as possible. Develop an eye for unsourced claims and consider why they are not forthcoming with the source. Draw your own independent conclusions from the raw data you collected. Have you noticed any of your freedoms slipping away? What are the benefits of "We the People" uniting together and preserving our freedoms while having the government serve the people?

9. *Destroying the family.* If there is a breakdown in the family, there is a *lack* of unity and strength in raising children on family terms. The children become elements of the court system and are immediately under *more control* of governing decisions. Each parent has a loss of rights in raising the child, and now the child is more likely to succumb more readily to the manipulation of others with an agenda, one of which is *not* in the child's best interest. The public school system is also free to manipulate children under government control at the lowest grade levels and has had decades to program them to their agenda. How could the influence of others program the minds of children? Who is trying to destroy family unity? What seems to be the reason for this happening? What appears to be its desired end result? How could this change things? Who does destroying the family unit benefit? Does the source for this breakdown appear

to have an agenda? Is the source overlooking, ignoring, or leaving out information that doesn't support its beliefs? Is the source using unnecessary language to sway the people's perception of the facts? How could the breakdown of the family be detrimental for "individuals" versus "the government"? How could a strong family unit strengthen the unity in a country? How could a strong family unit weaken the government? What effects do you see with the breakdown of the family? What type of unbiased research can be performed to find out more information? Find credible sources and gather as much information as possible. Research and then analyze all of the data collected. Formulate your own conclusions without prejudice.

10. *Destroying the churches.* Churches are units of strength with an image of morality or some sort of moral code. Each one may stand on its own ground and for possibly different things. Yet it is something that the government fears as it threatens its agenda. What would be the result of weakening or breaking down the unity of churches? Who is attempting to do this? What appears to be the desired end result of the disunity of the church? How would this change things? Who would benefit from this? How would this change the moral code of governing bodies? Does the source of this destruction appear to have an agenda? Is the source overlooking, ignoring, or leaving out information that doesn't support its agenda? Is the source using unnecessary influence to sway the people's perception of the facts? Where can you research using unbiased resources? What do different churches stand for? Why might the government be threatened by them? Who benefits from the strength and teachings of a church? Using credible sources, perform extensive research regarding this topic. Ask lots of questions and seek as much information as possible without prejudice. Evaluate, analyze, and draw your own independent conclusions.

11. *Taking over the educational system.* It is not an accident that government sources have taken over and monopolized *control* over the public school system and the *content* of information pushed onto the children and in universities. From the earliest stages of school life through college, and even in advanced education, the government has taken over control of education. By brainwashing vulnerable people willing to learn and absorb the information presented from whom they believe to be trusted sources, the political agenda has been advancing for generations. How are students in most educational systems being brainwashed and manipulated with an intentional agenda? What seems to be the reason for this happening? What appears to be the desired end results? How will this change things? Whom does this benefit? Why was God taken out of the public school system? Why are political agendas inserted into them? What is the premise of controlling the responses students give? How are opinions of students being controlled by the educational system? How might capturing the minds of children in the early years of education benefit the agenda of those who control the system? Is unnecessary language being used to persuade? How about in medical education? Do you notice any significant changes through the years? Who is funding large universities? Is information being left out or deceptive? How can you find unbiased research regarding this topic? What do you think is going on? Utilize the research gathered and formulate your own unbiased and independent conclusions.

It is vitally important to critically think about the ways manipulation can and will occur. There is no doubt that you are surrounded by propaganda and manipulation. Yet do not take my word for it; do your own independent and unbiased research and discover information from opposing sides. Formulate your own conclusions following adequate and thorough research. Find out where it takes you. Does any of it come as a surprise? What area has the greatest impact on you? Why do you think that is? What have you learned? How are you affected by this information?

Now that propaganda has been released like a "genie from a bottle," with *permission and encouragement to provide false information and misinformation to fit a predefined agenda*, there is no "putting it back" into the bottle. How does the propaganda in social media affect you, your patients, and your practice? Businesses? Other groups or organizations? How about Big Pharma and its new era of explicitly, politically, and carelessly promoting drugs and its agenda on all media sources now? Think about the fact that the information is *not required* to *be* factual. Did you previously know this? Are you concerned with these advertising and subliminal messages knowing the *permission to deceive*? How can you protect yourself and your patients or customers from false or altered-truth information? Who benefits from this information?

Imagine if society—rather than play into siding with emotional "group think," as desired and designed by the elite—worked together *in unity with one another*, supporting one another *for the good of our nation as a whole*. And what if we allowed the governing bodies to work for "We the People" rather than for "We the sheeple"?

There are so many questions to be asked and information to be verified. Be careful as you navigate the muddy (and often polluted) waters of propaganda, and remember to critically think and perform extensive independent research before formulating conclusions. And *never* forget that all media has been *permitted since 2013 to deceive, lie, and misinform*.

> *The most effective way to destroy people is to deny and obliterate their own understanding of their history.*
> —George Orwell

> *Propaganda is to a democracy what the bludgeon is to a totalitarian state.*
> —Noam Chomsky

MEDICALLY SPEAKING, WHO CONNECTS YOUR DOTS?

*You can sway a thousand men by appealing to their prejudices
quicker than you can convince one man by logic.*
—Robert A. Heinlein

*The whole aim of practical politics is to keep the population
alarmed (and hence clamorous to be led to safety) by an
endless series of hobgoblins, most of them imaginary.*
—H. L. Mencken

*Modern industrial civilization has developed within a certain
system of convenient myths. The driving force of modern
industrial civilization has been individual material gain, which
is accepted as legitimate, even praiseworthy, on the grounds that
private vices yield public benefits in the classic formulation.
Now, it's long been understood very well that a society that is based
on this principle will destroy itself in time. It can only persist with
whatever suffering and injustice it entails as long as it's possible to
pretend that the destructive forces that humans create are limited: that
the world is an infinite garbage can. At this stage of history, either
one of two things is possible: either the general population will take
control of its own destiny and will concern itself with community-
interests, guided by values of solidarity and sympathy and concern for
others; or, alternatively, there will be no destiny for anyone to control.
As long as some specialized class is in a position of authority, it is going
to set policy in the special interests that it serves. But the conditions
of survival, let alone justice, require rational social planning in the
interests of the community as a whole and, by now, that means the
global community. The question is whether privileged elites should
dominate mass-communication and should use this power as they
tell us they must, namely, to impose necessary illusions, manipulate
and deceive the stupid majority, and remove them from the public
arena. The question, in brief, is whether democracy and freedom
are values to be preserved or threats to be avoided. In this possibly
terminal phase of human existence, democracy and freedom are more
than values to be treasured, they may well be essential to survival.*
—Noam Chomsky

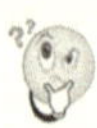

Reflect

1. How have you noticed changes in propaganda through the past five years? Ten? Thirty?
2. How does propaganda affect you? Your practice? Your patients, customers, career, or business?
3. How could propaganda be used to the benefit of the American people? How about to their detriment?
4. What is your biggest concern regarding the current status of drug propaganda in all of the major media sources, Big Tech, Big Pharma, and the like?
5. How will you evaluate information obtained from major news outlets, journalists, and so forth, knowing they have permission to lie and deceive? Will you change how you process this information?
6. How can critical thinking help sort through propaganda?
7. How will you evaluate or research information that you feel is concerning?
8. What other forms of manipulation can you add to the list included in this chapter? How would you critically think about the additional forms you came up with?
9. Read the books, cliff notes, or a summary of the books, plus the Act mentioned in this chapter. How do you see a correlation to where we are today? What other titles can you think of that have information regarding this topic?

———————

CHAPTER 7

Why Ban the Best?

According to research performed by the Front Line COVID-19 Critical Care (FLCCC) Alliance,[12] among others, ivermectin is one of the safest known drugs. It is on the World Health Organization's list of essential medicines, has been given over four billion times around the world, and has won the Nobel Prize for its global and historical impacts in eradicating endemic parasitic infections in many parts of the world. So *why* did "those in authority" ban the use of this drug when needed the most when presented with COVID-19? Who decided to ban it? Why did this source go so far as to "pursue" those who were writing, administering, or dispensing ivermectin? What seems to be the reason for this happening? What appears to be the desired end result of the ban? How could and did this ban impact people? Who benefited from the ban? Was there a financial incentive? Who suffered because of the ban? Did the source of the ban appear to have an agenda? Did the source overlook, ignore, or leave out information that didn't support its agenda? Did the source censor those who favored and promoted the healing effects of ivermectin? Why might they do this? Is the source a for-profit organization? Did the source use unnecessary language to instill fear or persuade the public's perception of the facts? Did the source try to manipulate the facts regarding the safety and efficacy of ivermectin? Did this safe drug mysteriously become unsafe overnight?

Be *objective* as you seek answers to these questions. Did the media outlets provide factual content or subjective and emotionally driven information? Did they appear biased or manipulative? Did they use fear as a motivating factor? Does it appear they may have been *linked* to the source of those who banned ivermectin? Now that you understand that the media is *not required to be factual*, how will you analyze this information? In addition, knowing the permission to lie, deceive, and manipulate for the sake of propaganda as per the Act signed in 2013, use your logical thinking to rationalize the use of "fact-checkers." Now that there is no moral guideline for the media to be truthful, is it ironic to use "fact-checkers" almost as a dramatic "comedy of errors," as even the so-called fact-checkers have no obligation to present the truth? What credentials do they even have? Hopefully, this is all starting to sink in—the vital necessity for each of you to do *your own* extensive research and draw *your own* logical conclusions.

The media has been blatantly clear regarding its position and has gone above and beyond to promote its for-profit and extremely prosperous agenda while censoring what does *not* fit its agenda, making it extremely difficult to see both sides of important issues. However, the information can be found if you are determined to deliberately "first do no harm" to your patients. To truly perform critical thinking methods, both sides of the issue must be researched in depth, evaluated, and analyzed before a conclusion is drawn by you alone without prejudice.

Approved for human use in 1987, ivermectin has been instrumental in tackling some of the world's most harmful tropical diseases, such as onchocerciasis, lymphatic filariasis (also known as elephantiasis), strongyloidiasis, and scabies.[13] It also effectively fights parasitic infestations in animals, which can be economically devastating to the livestock industry. In addition to being an effective, broad-spectrum antiparasitic, many healthcare professionals have been using ivermectin for decades to treat a variety of other diseases.

In 2017, according to Andy Crump in *The Journal of Antibiotics*, *"Few, if any, other drugs can rival ivermectin for its beneficial impact on human health and welfare."*[14] Crump worked for decades with

Satoshi Ōmura, the Japanese microbiologist responsible for *discovering* ivermectin.

Spend some time researching the names referenced previously and collecting additional information regarding ivermectin's safety and efficacy profile. How many times in your career have you dispensed, written for, or administered ivermectin? Were there any adverse effects? Did the drug prove to be effective? Suppose you haven't questioned the events surrounding the ban on ivermectin yet. In that case, *it's time to critically think* about why this safe and effective drug was forbidden for use when the recovery rate from the use of this drug is *astounding*. Do your own research using multiple, verified, and credible sources, and ask yourself these and many other questions.

The same holds true with hydroxychloroquine. When was the last time you dispensed this medication? What was the result? Was it effective? Was it safe? How many years has it been on the market? What is the safety history of this medication? Why was this drug banned from helping people who need it? Why were physicians censored, terminated, and eradicated from speaking out regarding the safety and efficacy of this historically successful drug? What does it say about these physicians who were willing to speak out with nothing to gain and no financial incentive, all in hopes of helping to improve or even save the lives of patients? What seemed to be the reason for this ban? Was it logical? What was the desired end result of the ban? Who did the ban benefit? Did the source of the ban appear to have an agenda? Was there a financial incentive attached to the ban? Why would "they" prohibit the use of a safe and helpful drug? Did the source overlook, ignore, or leave out information that didn't support its agenda? Did the source use unnecessary persuasion or manipulation to sway the people's perceptions? Was "the source" required to be truthful? Who was censored if they spoke up with an opposing view?

Research the safety and efficacy profiles of both ivermectin and hydroxychloroquine. Find numerous credible sources and collect raw data regarding these drugs. Without prejudice, analyze the data and evaluate the risk-versus-benefit profile regarding their use for combating the coronavirus, with improvements generally seen by day two with either drug. What do you conclude?

Refer to FLCCC.net as a potential source to find more information regarding the protocols used in the prevention and treatment of COVID-19 in both children and adults in numerous categories. Take note of the scientific evidence provided and shared openly. Taken from the FLCCC Alliance, "The Totality of Evidence" reads as follows:[15]

The Totality of Evidence

Decision-making in medicine can be difficult. The best decisions are based on a combination of the following:

1. The best available evidence
2. The clinician's experience, knowledge, and skills
3. The patient's individual circumstances, wants, and needs

Evidence can come in many forms: systematic reviews and meta-analyses (SRMAs), randomized controlled trials (RCTs), observational controlled trials (OCTs), epidemiological analyses, case series, and patient anecdotes.

For a long time, RCTs were considered the "gold standard" of evidence. In this type of clinical trial, participants are randomly assigned to either a treatment group or a control group. You may have heard the term RCT with reference to the various medications being considered as possible COVID-19 treatments.

Another term you may have heard is "meta-analysis" or SRMA. SRMAs involve systematically reviewing the published literature to combine patient data (qualitative and quantitative) from numerous studies of a particular medical intervention to reach a conclusion that has greater statistical power than any single study. Because of the methodology of combining data from multiple studies, SRMAs look at an increased number of subjects, with greater diversity among subjects, and can identify accumulated effects.

However, both RCTs and SRMAs can suffer from the same flaws as other study designs, and, unfortunately, these flaws are sometimes intentional due to the financial influences on both researchers and journal editors.

For example, SRMAs can lead to inaccurate results because of biased inclusion or exclusion of study data, flawed analyses, or the exclusion of unpublished studies.

The problems with RCTs are numerous, not least of which is the heavy influence of the pharmaceutical industry in the design and execution of studies, particularly in the larger, well-funded studies published in high-impact medical journals. *Studies can be designed to produce a particular set of results, and often are,* so much so that often RCTs *do not accurately reflect* real-world clinical impacts.

"It is simply no longer possible to believe much of the clinical research that is published, or to rely on the judgment of trusted physicians or authoritative medical guidelines," wrote Dr. Marcia Angell, in her book *The Truth About Drug Companies: How They Deceive Us and What to Do About It.* *"I take no pleasure in this conclusion, which I reached slowly and reluctantly over my two decades as an*

editor of the New England Journal of Medicine (NEJM)," she continued.

Angell wrote that medical journals have become *"primarily a marketing machine to sell drugs of dubious benefit,"* and suggested that the pharmaceutical industry has so much wealth and power that it is able to co-opt any institution that might stand in its way. This, she says, includes Congress, the FDA, academic medical centers, *"and the medical profession itself."*

Angell and her husband, Arthur Reiman—a Harvard professor who also edited NEJM for decades—warned of the undue influence of the pharmaceutical industry for years, as did many other doctors, researchers, and medical ethicists.

"The case against science is straightforward: much of the scientific literature, perhaps half, may simply be untrue… In their quest for telling a compelling story, scientists too often sculpt data to fit their preferred theory of the world. Or they retro-fit hypotheses to fit their data," Richard Horton, Editor-in-Chief of *The Lancet*, wrote in 2015.

In 2005, Stanford professor John P. Ioannidis wrote an article entitled *Why Most Published Research Findings are False*, stating, "It *is more likely for a research claim to be false than true. Moreover, for many current scientific fields, claimed research findings may often be simply accu-rate measures of the prevailing bias."*

In a 2014 paper, Ioannidis analyzed over nine thousand published meta-analyses in bio-medicine and found that *one in five was flawed beyond repair. Another one in three was redundant and unnecessary*, while many others were decent but had "noninformative" evidence. Good and truly informative meta-analyses, he found, were a small minority *(three percent)*.

An analysis in 2011 looked at the overall quality of evidence behind forty-one guidelines put out by the Infectious Disease Society of America between 1994 and 2010. Only *fourteen percent* of the guidelines were based on the supposed "gold standard" of RCTs. Nearly *forty percent* were based on *expert opinion alone*. So where, you might ask, does that leave us when it comes to decision-making in healthcare?

A New Model: Weighing Up All the Evidence

Just as a jury is asked to review and evaluate all the evidence put forth during a trial, so too must clinicians look at all the best available evidence before them. It is proposed that researchers rely on the *"totality of evidence"* and incorporate data from basic science, pharmacology, epidemiology, clinical experience, OTCs, RCTs, and SRMAs.

A common type of observational study is an OCT, where investigators *retrospectively* assess health outcomes among groups of participants according to a research plan or protocol. The outcomes of study subjects receiving medical interventions (such as drugs, devices, or procedures) are compared to the outcomes of subjects that did not. In these comparisons, the subjects are not randomly assigned to specific interventions by the investigator (as in a prospective RCT). Many discount the value of findings from OCTs due to an excessive concern that the results can be incorrectly interpreted due to the existence of unmeasured confounders, such as certain characteristics or the behavior of both the patients and the treating physicians.

Although such concerns are valid when relying on the results of a single OCT, the reality is that findings based on data from groups of OCTs are, on average, *identical* to the findings from groups of RCTs. Unfortunately, in modern medicine, this fact is rarely taught to, or appreciated by, physicians and researchers.

"The whole art of medicine is in observation," said Dr. William Osler, a Canadian physician often described as the father of modern medicine.

A study published in 2014 looked at healthcare outcomes assessed with observational study designs compared with those assessed with randomized trials. The researchers reported, *"On average, there is little evidence for significant effect to estimate differences between observational studies and RCTs, regardless of specific observational study design, heterogeneity, or inclusion of studies of pharmacological interventions."*

The American Thoracic Society (ATS), in an official 2020 research statement said, *"Observational studies can provide evidence in representative and diverse patient populations. Quality observational studies should be sought in the development of ATS clinical practice guidelines, and in medical decision-making."*

The Totality of Evidence for Ivermectin in COVID-19

Based on the preceding, it is important to look at evidence from all sources when deciding whether to use a particular treatment approach. FLCCC used the *totality of evidence* approach when deciding on whether to recommend ivermectin as a potential treatment for COVID-19.

Some examples of the evidence they looked at include the following (not an exhaustive list):

- Basic science:
  - o The FDA-approved drug ivermectin inhibits the replication of SARS-CoV-2 in vitro
  - o The broad spectrum antiviral ivermectin *targets* the host nuclear transport importin $\alpha/\beta 1$ heterodimer Ivermectin inhibits DNA polymerase UL42 of pseudorabies virus entrance into the nucleus and proliferation of the virus in vitro and vivo
  - o Ivermectin is a potent inhibitor of flavivirus replication specifically targeting NS3 helicase activity: new prospects for an old drug
  - o Nuclear localization of dengue virus (DENV) 1–4 non-structural protein 5; protection against all 4 DENV serotypes by the inhibitor Ivermectin
  - o Inhibition of Human Adenovirus Replication by the Importin $\alpha/\beta 1$ Nuclear Import Inhibitor Ivermectin
- Pharmacology:
  - o Ivermectin Docks to the SARS-CoV-2 Spike Receptor-binding Domain Attached to ACE2
  - o Coronavirus (2019-nCoV) Deactivation via Spike Glycoprotein Shielding by Old Drugs, Bioinformatic Study

- o Clinical Trial Conducted by MedinCell Confirms the Safety of Continuous Administration of Ivermectin
- o Avermectin exerts an anti-inflammatory effect by downregulating the nuclear transcription factor kappa-B and mitogen-activated protein kinase activation pathway
- o Ivermectin inhibits LPS-induced production of inflammatory cytokines and improves LPS-induced survival in mice
- o Effect of ivermectin on the cellular and humoral immune responses of rabbits
- Epidemiology:
  - o Uttar Pradesh government says early use of Ivermectin helped to keep positivity, deaths low
  - o Sharp Reductions in COVID-19 Case Fatalities and Excess Deaths in Peru in Close Time Conjunction, State-By-State, with Ivermectin Treatments
  - o Ivermectin: Partial monitoring results provided in extended use in positive patients (Argentina)
- Observational studies:
  - o Regular Use of Ivermectin as Prophylaxis for COVID-19 Led Up to a 92% Reduction in COVID-19 Mortality Rate in a Dose-Response Manner: Results of a Prospective Observational Study of a Strictly Controlled Population of 88,012 Subjects
  - o Use of Ivermectin Is Associated with Lower Mortality in Hospitalized Patients with Coronavirus Disease 2019

- o Ivermectin as Pre-exposure Prophylaxis for COVID-19 among Healthcare Providers in a Selected Tertiary Hospital in Dhaka—An Observational Study
  - o Why COVID-19 is not so spread in Africa: How does Ivermectin affect it?
- Randomized controlled trials:
  - o Use of Ivermectin as a Potential Chemoprophylaxis for COVID-19 in Egypt: A Randomized Clinical Trial
  - o Role of ivermectin in the prevention of SARS-CoV-2 infection among health-care workers in India: A matched case-control study
- Systematic Reviews and Meta-Analyses:
  - o Review of the Emerging Evidence Demonstrating the Efficacy of Ivermectin in the Prophylaxis and Treatment of COVID-19 (this study was what is called a "narrative review.")
  - o Ivermectin for Prevention and Treatment of COVID-19 Infection: A Systematic Review, Meta-analysis, and Trial Sequential Analysis to Inform Clinical Guidelines
- Case Series:
  - o The Use of Compassionate Ivermectin in the Management of Symptomatic Outpatients and Hospitalized Patients with Clinical Diagnosis of COVID-19 at the Centro Medico Bournigal and at the Centro Medico Punta Cana, Grupo Rescue, Dominican Republic, from May 1

Further studies continue to look at the use of ivermectin in COVID-19. A full analysis of all studies is available at c19ivermectin.com, and a real-time meta-analysis is found at ivmmeta.com. You can also read the work of researchers such as Alexandros Marinos *(Do Your Own Research)* and Phil Harper *(The Digger)* or follow Dr. Pierre Kory's writings about ivermectin and Big Pharma *(Pierre Kory's Medical Musings)*.

Video:
   A Drug's Efficacy is Determined by Looking at the "Totality of Evidence"

While ivermectin is a remarkably safe drug with minimal adverse reactions (almost all minor), some potential drug interactions should be reviewed before prescribing ivermectin. The most important drug–drug interactions occur with cyclosporin, tacrolimus, antiretroviral drugs, and certain antifungal drugs.

As a medical clinician, it is important to think critically and question the validity and credibility of information. As you can see in the information provided, it is more important now than ever to verify your sources and research many different ones, as false or "misinformation" is becoming more and more prevalent. Understand that *even drug companies themselves* may *not* be providing true and accurate information. Keep in mind that they are "for profit" and possess a definite financial incentive tied to their output. *Follow the money.* You will find that the people, sites, and writings referenced here are financially incentive-free, with nothing to gain other than the sharing of pertinent information from one professional to another, with the goal of *best treatment practices* for the patient.

Beware of ignorance when in motion; look out for inexperience when in action and beware of the majority when mentally poisoned with misinformation, for collective ignorance does not become wisdom.
   —William J. H. Boetcker

MEDICALLY SPEAKING, WHO CONNECTS YOUR DOTS?

*At any given moment, public opinion is a chaos of
suspicion, misinformation, and prejudice.*
—Gore Vidal

*If you repeat a lie often enough, people will believe it. It
really is public brainwashing and misinformation.*
—Robert Kane Pappas

*The lowest form of popular culture—lack of information,
misinformation, disinformation, and a contempt for the truth or
the reality of most people's lives—has overrun real journalism.*
—Carl Bernstein

*Nothing can now be believed which is seen in a newspaper.
Truth itself becomes suspicious by being put into that polluted
vehicle. The real extent of this state of misinformation
is known only to those who are in situations to confront
facts within their knowledge with the lies of the day.*
—Thomas Jefferson

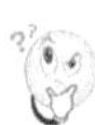

Reflect

1. Based on your own observation of ivermectin use, what
   conclusions do you draw regarding its safety and efficacy
   profile? What additional sources can you research to deny
   or affirm your claim? Use critical thinking in your analysis.
2. How can you incorporate more critical thinking and less
   influential distractions into your decisions regarding drug
   safety and efficacy?
3. Evaluate your research regarding the safety and efficacy of
   ivermectin and hydroxychloroquine, and consider why you
   think these drugs were banned from therapy for COVID-

19 patients. Run this question through the critical thinking process.

4. What surprised you the most regarding the accuracy, or lack thereof, of medical information and data being presented by reputable journals and drug companies? What are your thoughts on their permission to lie, deceive, and manipulate? How will you proceed to extract, analyze, and use relevant drug information in the future? Where will you go for credible resources? Critically think about each resource you select.

CHAPTER 8

Vaxed or Vexed?

By now, the media and Big Pharma's version of the "vaccine" has been made known. They have been intent on showing one side only and censoring *anyone* who presents with an opposing view. Why is that? Does that make you think about what they may be hiding? What are the reasons someone might censor someone else?

In this country, there is a right to freedom of speech; therefore, how is it even logical or legal to *censor* someone else? As a critical thinker, it is time to consider an opposing side to this topic. In this case, look at it from a *nonprofit* perspective—from those who have nothing to gain from this product and have actually lost because of speaking out regarding what they *personally* saw firsthand. The viewpoint that has been made public on major media outlets is a "for profit," financially incentivized vantage point, funded by the drug companies themselves, as you may or may not have known.

What were some of the safety features "they" (Big Pharma) promised regarding the injection? According to a declaration treaty signed by seventeen thousand doctors and scientists[16] (and counting), including the presenter, Dr. Michael Yeadon, and with additional input from Dr. Kelly Victory[17] and Dr. Ryan Cole,[18, 19] the following concerns have become known:

1. *They "claimed" that toxic spike proteins would remain in the deltoid at the injection site.* This is proven *false*. Rather,

they are *widely* distributed throughout the *entire* body. Humans are being used as an mRNA platform. This has *never* happened before. The injection causes the expression in the human body of *toxic spike proteins*, widely distributed, leading to toxicity. The mRNA goes *anywhere* and *everywhere* in the body, producing spike proteins, which induce inflammation. The spike proteins form in both white and gray matter, including binding in muscles and capillary vessels. People who have been injected are now a *"little factory producing gobs of toxic proteins in every organ system in the body. The vaccine causes you to produce the same precise toxic spike proteins with no off switch,"* says Dr. Kelly Victory,[20] a board-certified trauma and emergency specialist. *"You now have the genetic machine to produce the spikes in every system of the body."* This causes *clotting*, among other things. Spike proteins bind to cancer cells and specific receptors, allowing them to grow and become *more prolific*. This could lead and has led to *new-onset cancers*. Since the injections, there has been an *uptick in cancers*, stated Dr. Ryan Cole,[21,22] a leading pathologist and immunology and virology expert. There has also been an *uptick in the Epstein-Barr virus, endometrial cancers, the growth of tumors*, and even *increased cell activity* in general. Deposited spike protein can become prolific, even resulting in *foot-long blood clots*. These clots are different from normal clots, states Dr. Ryan Cole, as they are *devoid* of hemoglobin, K^+, and Fe^{+2}, *not* the typical blood clots. The clotting has presented itself as *heart attacks, strokes,* and *blood clots to the lungs*, among other maladies. Spike proteins lead to *clotting diseases; endothelial diseases*. Postmortem, these fibrous clots present an unusual amount of collected proteins, including *fibrin, amyloid, sugars, and glycoproteins*, making them *elastic*. The body does not easily break down amyloid. This is an entirely *new* type of clot.

2. *They "claimed" that the mRNA would be eliminated quickly.* This is proven *false*. The mRNA *continues to proliferate*

throughout *every* organ system in the human body, even *affecting eggs and sperm*, negatively affecting normal processes. There is an inhibition of neurons in the ovary itself, *decreasing fertility*. Placentas have been shown to be calcified, including spike proteins, and inducing excess inflammation. Evidence of the spike protein is found even *longer than twelve months past* the injection date.

3. *They "claimed" it couldn't be incorporated into the DNA.* This is proven *false* as well. As mentioned previously, it is prolific and has been *distributed throughout* the entire body. They are "immune imprinting." There has been an injection of the gene sequence.

4. *There is evidence of questionable practices all around.* Several studies were clearly *unblinded* while they were ongoing. This is *against* best practice. In several cases, subjects were *removed* from the database *prior to* the statistical analysis in a way suggestive of *fraud*. The public was given blanket assurances time and again by *all* of the companies (Pfizer, Moderna, BioNTech, Janssen, and Astra-Zeneca, in addition to their enablers) about the "benign" safety profile of their products, even as the products rolled out in the earliest weeks, knowing this was *not true*.

5. *The packaging is highly comprised of omissions of standard safety studies.* Even the packaging does *not* include the fact that the mRNA *does* leave the injection site while they told the public it doesn't. They *have not conducted* complete reproductive toxicology studies, without which the injection should *never* be given to pregnant women. Not all the components have been through toxicity testing.

6. *The "vaccine" provides little to no protection from the virus.* Dr. Ryan Cole discussed that HIV also mutates, just like the coronavirus. That is why there is no vaccine for HIV. It is peculiar that something was created for the coronavirus with the same mutational characteristics as HIV.

7. *There is no risk or age population defined.* According to Dr. Ryan Cole, this is the *only* "vaccine" *ever* not to do this.

8. *This "vaccine" did not go through the proper protocol.* Gene-based products usually go through five to ten years of study. This product did *not* go through gene mutation studies. The product displays adverse effects from modulation as time goes by. Dr. Ryan Cole also presented the well-known statement, *"If you see something, say something."* As countless doctors have been seeing things in their particular practices, such as pathology, virology, epidemiology, internal medicine, cardiology, and morticians and embalmers, they have also tried to "say something." Yet they have been censored, penalized, terminated, or in some way silenced. Why might this be? Keep in mind, according to the Act passed in 2013, propaganda allows lies, deception, and even misinformation. Therefore, censorship is not based on any of these factors, if any had come into play. So, what other reasons could there be for censorship? Again, as stated by Dr. Ryan Cole, *"The cells don't lie."* He and the other doctors and clinicians included in the bibliography have presented what they have *personally* seen and witnessed as displayed by the cells themselves.

9. *No informed consent was obtained.* Medical clinicians have written for, dispensed, and/or administered this product without *"informed"* consent or knowledge of pertinent facts. These people had a *right to know* the truth behind the product rather than a harmful, sometimes even fatal, deception. Most medical professionals have *not* been informed of this information, especially when the product was initially presented for use. They had to rely on the *claims* made by Big Pharma through major media outlets. Big Pharma and the media went so far as to censor any other information that was brought forth in good faith. In addition, patients and customers had *not*, and have *not*, been presented with "informed" consent as well.

The same seventeen thousand doctors and scientists claim, *"We declare that Pfizer, Moderna, BioNTech, Janssen, Astra-Zeneca, and their enablers withheld, and willfully omitted, safety and effectiveness information from patients, and physicians, and should be immediately indicted for fraud.*"[23] The claim was read by Michael Yeadon, Ph.D., the former vice president and chief science officer of the Allergy and Respiratory Research for Pfizer Inc.

Take some time and do *your own* research. Ask yourself, if even one small part of the information presented in this chapter is true, what could this mean to you, your family, your patients, or anyone who conceded to receiving this injection *without full disclosure* of safety and efficacy information? And if you are *resistant* to open your mind to the possibility that any portion of this may be true, ask yourself, Why? What research are you standing by? Are you choosing to willfully put the lives of your patients in jeopardy under your care and guidance now that you've seen additional data? Who performed the research? Are you open to reviewing new research as it arises? What ties do "they" have to for-profit organizations?

Recall the Act written in 2013 regarding propaganda and the right to lie, deceive, and falsify information to promote propagation. If you determine that any or all of this research presented here may be true and the information provided reveals that the body of those injected has become a "spike protein factory," working nonstop and consistently making more, what could the consequences be? *Would it be wise to seek a way to try to stop these spike protein factories?* What might happen if you avoided the issue and allowed the factories to continue to produce spike proteins throughout the body?

What do you know about spike proteins? What resources will you use to find out more information? Take time to understand what spike proteins are, how they are formed, and their effect on the human body. Is this something you want in yourself, a loved one, a patient, or a customer? The human body's cells were *not made* for foreign spike proteins.

Jeff Childers presents a fun and sarcastic daily news summary regarding the latest COVID updates in his newsletter found at coffeeandcovid.com. Theepochtimes.com also has information that can be reviewed. Dr. Peter A. McCullough[24]—a cardiologist, internist, epidemiologist, professor of medicine, one of the top five most-published medical researchers in the United States, and editor of two medical journals—questioned the lack of vax safety data.[25]

In his findings, the vax causes spike protein to linger in the body, even *greater than twelve months, weakening the immune system.* And that's opposed to the false claim of the proteins being eliminated immediately. He went on to report vaccine-related injuries and deaths. He is well-known for his research and input into what he has *seen* and *experienced firsthand,* as well as his censorship and banning for *"if you see something, say something."* Dr. McCullough has proposed a treatment algorithm as an early treatment protocol, now known as the *McCullough Protocol 2022.* Take some time to review this strategy. He has also defined a vitamin and supplement protocol to be included in the early treatment stages as supportive therapies. Research these experts on your own to find out more information.

Dr. Robert Malone discussed information regarding mRNA from vaccines.[26] Who is Dr. Malone? He is an internationally recognized scientist and physician and the original *inventor of mRNA vaccination* as a technology, *DNA vaccination,* and multiple *nonviral DNA and RNA/mRNA platform delivery* technologies. He holds numerous fundamental domestic and foreign patents in the fields of gene delivery, delivery formulations, and vaccines, including fundamental DNA and RNA/mRNA vaccine technologies. Dr. Malone states the following regarding his current pursuits:

> *It started with my own experiences and concerns regarding the safety and bioethics of how the COVID-19 genetic vaccines were developed and forced upon the world, and then expanded as I discovered the many short-cuts, database issues, obfuscation and frankly, lies told in the development of the spike protein-based genetic vaccines for SARS-CoV-2. Personal experiences involving identifying, developing, and trying to publish peer-reviewed academic papers focused on drug repurposing and the rights of physicians to practice medicine as well as what I have seen close colleagues go through have*

> *further influenced me. Finally, as unethical man-*
> *dates for administering experimental vaccines to*
> *adults and children began to be pushed by govern-*
> *ments, my research into what I believe is author-*
> *itarian control by governments that are being*
> *manipulated by large corporations (big finance,*
> *big pharmaceutical, big media and big technology)*
> *influenced my changing world view.*

As a virologist, Dr. Malone has spent most of his career work-ing on vaccine development. He has also had extensive experience in drug repurposing for infectious disease outbreaks. Regarding the clinical trials for the mRNA vaccines, he states,

> *These trials must have had their pre-clinical*
> *data packages signed off on, which means that all of*
> *the adverse events, mRNA stability issues, and the*
> *nanolipid particle issues in the original pre-clinical*
> *data package must have been "normalized" by the*
> *FDA. Because frankly, there has not been enough*
> *time to run pre-clinical trials on all of these vaccine*
> *candidates. Please go to* clinicaltrials.gov *and do a*
> *search on mRNA vaccines. What has happened over*
> *the last two years has me questioning everything*
> *that the FDA has done and is doing. All indications*
> *are that the administrative state that runs the FDA*
> *has been corrupted by pharma.*

Find out more about Dr. Malone at rwmalonemd.com. He has also authored the book *Lies My Gov't Told Me: And the Better Future Coming.*

With all this information, especially being known by these companies and the media from the very beginning, you should ask yourself why the media was adamant about delivering a message that the vaccine will only work if *everyone* gets it. What is the logic behind this? Why were the other medications *suppressed*, such as *hydroxy-*

chloroquine and *ivermectin*, while forcing a *redirected focus* toward the *vaccine* instead? Was there an attempt to inject *everyone* with gene-altering spike proteins, *weakening the entire human population*? Why were there different "versions" of the injections? Were the ones the "elites" were shown to have been given really "COVID vaccines" as well? Or could they have been placebos? And now that *billions* of people have been injected with one, two, three, four, and in some people, even five or more injections of spike proteins, is it ironic that the ban on safe and effective medications taken orally has *suddenly* lessened? Have the safety profiles of hydroxychloroquine and ivermectin mysteriously been "rediscovered," showing them safe and effective *once again* as they *always* were? *Has the damage already been done?*

Have you noticed any peculiar instances of "sudden adult death syndrome" from athletes and supposedly otherwise young and healthy individuals? Take some time to watch the documentary titled *Died Suddenly 2022 (Full Documentary).*[27] What are your thoughts on possible causes? Why did Anthony Fauci *discourage autopsies* on patients who received vaccines? Was there something to hide, such as *spike protein "elastic" clots?*

Take some time and explore autopsy results recorded by hundreds of coroners, pathologists, morticians, embalmers, and so forth in this documentary. Research as much as possible and gather your own data from an unprejudiced standpoint. The media has been clear on what information they want the world to know. Now, take some time to do *your own* research on an opposing side and see what you may uncover.

In your field of patient care, it is always vital to *first, do no harm.* Sometimes this may entail doing extra research as new information presents itself and finding the facts for yourself. Evaluate carefully all the information you collect. Ask yourself dozens of questions regarding your findings. Process *all* of the information through the critical thinking guidelines presented in earlier chapters. With this topic alone, there will be more and more information developing daily. Have an open mind and collect as much information as possible so you may make an informed and logical conclusion on your own.

*Censorship no longer works by hiding information from
you; censorship works by flooding you with immense
amounts of misinformation, of irrelevant information,
of funny cat videos, until you are unable to focus.*
—Yuval Noah Harari

*I have said that propaganda, misinformation and disinformation
have always been part of political warfare. Social media and
other new platforms have given it a new life and reach through
which the fake news phenomenon can reach everywhere.*
—Bilawal Bhutto Zardari

*At any given moment, public opinion is a chaos of
superstition, misinformation and prejudice.*
—Gore Vidal

*Until we have a better relationship between private performance
and the public truth, as was demonstrated with Watergate, we as the
public are absolutely right to remain suspicious, contemptuous even,
of the secrecy and the misinformation which is the digest of our news.*
—John le Carré

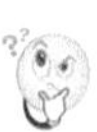

Reflect

1. What is your current position regarding the COVID-19 "vaccine"? What sources of information have you used to reach this conclusion? Name factors that have affected how you made your decisions.
2. Are you able to place all biases aside and critically think about both sides of this issue? If so, what resources will you begin with? If not, what is the basis for your bias?
3. How can you incorporate more critical thinking and less influential distractions into the decisions?

4. What research presented in this chapter surprised you the most? What have you learned from it? Will it change the way you view media coverage? Will it change how you practice?

5. Take some time to *follow the money.* Then, compare potential motives behind Big Pharma and the media versus those of the seventeen-thousand-plus clinical professionals presenting their findings, many of whom actually *lost* things, such as positions or their platforms, in doing so.

6. Are there news sources you can find that are *not* persuading you to choose one side or another or just want to share facts for the sake of information?

7. Describe your thoughts on spike proteins and the factories that have been created in every system in the bodies of those injected. Have you personally experienced a concern regarding the infiltration of spike proteins?

8. While the past cannot be undone, how can you move forward in helping with a *solution* or *resolution* to this or other new medical issues? How can you further protect, guide, and do no harm to your patients?

CHAPTER 9

Why Censor?

> *Censorship is the suppression of speech, public communication, or other information. Political censorship exists when a government attempts to conceal, fake, distort, or falsify information that its citizens receive by suppressing or crowding out political news that the public might receive through news outlets.*

People are unable to dissent from the government or political party in charge in the absence of neutral or objective information. This is something they count on.

> *This term also extends to the systematic suppression of views that are contrary to those of the government in power. The government often possesses the power of the army and the secret police, to enforce the compliance of journalists with the will of the authorities to spread the story that the ruling authorities want the people to believe. At times this involves bribery, defamation, imprisonment, and even assassination.*[28]

There are many different forms of censorship found in many different arenas. Even self-censorship is sometimes used by authors, artists, inventors, and the like to protect their artistic work. It is important not only to be aware that censorship exists but also to be able to critically think through each case of censorship you may encounter. You need to be able to draw your own conclusions based on *logic and sound reasoning* backed by evidence and raw data. Lacking the ability to think critically could be detrimental to your ability to come to a truth-based conclusion. You must possess the ability to analyze information effectively and without prejudice.

Your "freedoms" in society today are disappearing faster than at any other time in history. There is a risk at hand if you do not learn to think more critically. There is a greater chance that you will succumb to fraud, manipulation, gaslighting, propaganda, and the like if you cannot think critically. Is there any evidence of censorship that you see in society today? Analyze the issue of censorship and all facts, data, and evidence related to it. The challenge is to do so without the influence of personal feelings, opinions, or biases. Analyze based on factual information only.

Once again, go back to the Act passed in 2013, permitting and encouraging false, deceptive, and mis- or disinformation in propaganda. As mentioned earlier, having read or listened to this, you now know that the censorship by the major news and social media outlets is *not* due to any form of misinformation since this was approved in 2013. Simply put, censorship is about *fear*; fear that *others will find out.*

Therefore, what are they afraid of? What don't they want *you* to know? The truth? Why are they censoring some of the *most intelligent* and *talented* people in the world for speaking out about what they personally witnessed in their fields of expertise? Any form of censorship, other than personal censorship to protect your own artistic work, should *raise a flag of alert* and make you desire to *seek additional information*, including extensive research regarding opposing views of the topic at hand. Censorship is based on the *insecurity* of the one doing the censoring. It is a fear of someone revealing something the *censor* doesn't want others to know. This should *always* make you begin the process of critical thinking.

Who is doing the censoring? What seems to be the reason for the censoring? What appears to be its desired end result? How could this change things? Who does the censoring benefit? Does the source of censoring appear to have an agenda? Is it emotionally driven? Is the source of the censoring overlooking, ignoring, or leaving out information that doesn't support its beliefs or claims? That particular question reveals censoring right there. Is the source of the censoring using unnecessary language to sway an audience's perception of a fact? Does *following the money* lead back to "the source"? *What are they hiding?*

Remember, your ability to *independently research* is key to having authenticity. Verify your source of information and evaluate it within your own means. If sources you discover are *unwilling* to expose *where* the information came from, let that be a red flag to you. Verify your sources. If possible, evaluate claims from both sides of an argument, being aware of possible biases from either or both sides. Practice setting aside your own biases, as this will most likely cloud your judgment. Learn to see things from alternate vantage points.

Do you identify censorship in the news media outlets today? How about in social media? How about in the entertainment industry? What about in the government or politics in general? How about on a local level in your community? Where else do you see censorship occurring? Have you ever censored anyone from anything? Has anyone ever censored you personally?

Critically think about the reasons behind each of the scenarios mentioned. Ask objective and unbiased questions. Always select the most important and relevant information regarding the topic, and in this case, censorship. Determine what is establishing a clear direction in what you are trying to figure out. What is your end goal? When you identify censoring, be *deliberate* and discover what the one being censored has to say. Find out as much as possible about *both* sides of the issue. Once you have gathered and collected the most relevant materials, assess the information and draw your own conclusions based on the unbiased data. This is such an important skill in mastering the art of critical thinking. What have you concluded about censorship? How do you see it in your surrounding environment? Be aware of the occurrences, and critically think in each case.

Censorship is to art as lynching is to justice.
—Henry Louis Gates Jr.

Whoever would overthrow the liberty of a nation
must begin by subduing the freeness of speech.
—Benjamin Franklin

Let us be clear: censorship is cowardice. It masks corruption. It is
a school of torture: it teaches and accustoms one to the use of force
against an idea, to submit thought to an alien "other." But worst still,
censorship destroys criticism, which is the essential ingredient of culture.
—Pablo Antonio Cuadra

"Once a government is committed to the principle of silencing the voice
of opposition, it has only one way to go, and that is down the path of
increasingly repressive measures, until it becomes a source of terror to
all its citizens and creates a country where everyone lives in fear.
—Harry S. Truman

Think for yourselves and let others enjoy the privilege to do so, too.
—Voltaire

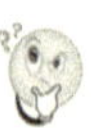

Reflect

1. Where do you notice censorship in the world today? How has it affected your practice?
2. Why have well-renowned clinicians been censored by media outlets? What do the media outlets fear? What are they afraid you may find out? What are your thoughts about

these clinicians being censored for speaking out regarding their findings?

3. Summarize the key elements of censorship. What conclusions do you draw?

4. How does the idea of censorship compare and contrast to the culture you live in today? Did you realize it has nothing to do with misinformation, as they claim?

5. What sources did you use to evaluate the censorship? What information did you see as most relevant?

6. What is your biggest concern regarding the conclusions you came to regarding censorship? What is the premise of your concern?

7. How will you use this information in your daily life? How does it affect you?

CHAPTER 10

Why Cancel?

Cancel culture, also known as call-out culture, is a phrase contemporary to the late two thousand tens to two thousand twenties used to refer to a culture in which those who are deemed to have acted or spoken in an unacceptable manner are ostracized, boycotted or shunned. This shunning may extend to social or professional circles—whether on social media or in person—with most high-profile incidents involving celebrities. Those subject to this ostracism are said to have been "canceled."[29]

"Canceling" can also be in the form of *publicly shaming* a person or group of people. It could also mean withdrawing support for some form of public figure or company based on something they did or said that was found to be in some way "offensive" or objectionable. It is a form of rejection that potentially denies someone the right to apologize or somehow resolve a mistake that may have been made. Whether a mistake or simply being objectionable, the possibility of being "called out" exists within the terms of the "cancel culture."

"Canceling" also stems from issues of *insecurity* and a *deep-seated need for control.* It is a version of "stomping your feet" to get your way and denying someone the right to their opinion or freedom of speech. Apply the same measures of critical thinking to the issues involving "cancel culture." What is the source of information? Where did it come from? Was it independently verified? How do you evaluate the source of information? How about the content of the information? What is the reliability of the source and the content? Do you fully understand the information collected? What additional resources have been used for interpretation?

What is the premise of the argument for canceling? Who stands to benefit from it? Who is doing what regarding canceling? What seems to be the goal or end result of the canceling? How could this change things? What was the position of the one being canceled? What appeared to be the premise? Evaluate the claims on both sides of the argument. View things from differing points of view. Does the source of canceling appear to have an agenda? Is it overlooking or intentionally leaving out information that opposes its claim? Is it using unnecessary language to sway the audience to its cancel? What does it fear from the one being "canceled"?

Assess the information regarding the canceling issue independently, extrapolating and discovering potential outcomes. Make a conscious effort to remain unbiased and use only relevant information based on confirmed and trusted sources. Using logical reasoning based on factual information, what do you think is going on?

How is "canceling" linked to conformity? Is it yet another method to snatch away your freedom? How do you perceive it in relation to a form of control? Realize that those who do the canceling are the ones who are afraid, insecure, and are trying to bully their way to power and control. They do not want you to think for yourself and especially express your own opinion if it differs from theirs. Understanding the source and the reasoning allows you to see more clearly when this is happening, by whom, and why.

Continue to utilize the same methods of critical thinking presented in this book. Train yourself to analyze situations using an array of relevant, factual, and unbiased sources, looking at them from opposing perspectives. Is the process of critical thinking becoming easier? Have you noticed yourself asking the same form of questions almost instinctively yet? Take the time to program this information into your mind so you become *automatically* programmed to think critically and instinctively regarding all matters.

In a cancel culture, we appoint ourselves the arbiters of
right and wrong and also the judge and jury, because
thanks to social media, we get to dole out punishment.
—Unknown

Cancel culture is not actually about justice. It is about control.
People use cancellation to force conformity to ideals.
—Teal Swan

Cancel culture is a pretentious form of bullying.
—Unknown

Cancel culture is a term bounced around by people
afraid of accountability. But freedom of speech
does not mean freedom from consequences.
—Monisha Rajesh

Cancel culture grows because we accept (and gluttonously
consume) social violence. We no longer seek truth or
both sides of a story. Whichever side is loudest, wins…
regardless of its relationship to the truth.
—Steve Maraboli

We live in a generation of emotionally weak people. Everything has
to be watered down because it's offensive, including the truth.
—Unknown

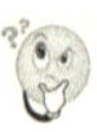

Reflect

1. Where do you notice cancel culture in the world today? How does it affect you? Have you ever been "canceled" because of your medical views?
2. Summarize the key elements of the cancel culture. What information do you draw from this?
3. How does the idea of cancel culture compare and contrast to the culture you live in today?
4. What sources did you use to evaluate the cancel culture? What information do you see as most relevant?
5. What is your biggest concern regarding your conclusions about cancel culture today? What is the premise of your concern?

CHAPTER 11

Why Identify?

Let me begin by saying that this chapter is meant in no way to place judgment upon anyone but rather to apply critical thinking methods regarding the desire to have a label placed on yourself to "identify" whatever that label may be.

In today's society, some people have become enraptured with labeling themselves with one aspect of their being. Why has it become so important to pick out one of many attributes and tag themselves with that regard? Everyone is beautifully and wonderfully made. We have talents, ambitions, gifts, and magnificent abilities. Why is there a "strong desire" to overlook a multitude of endearing and even impressive qualities just to focus on a decision to think a particular thought and label oneself with this "identity"? More importantly, how did this become a *movement* and take flight to the point that our very own government now finds it necessary to create mandates regarding this desire to highlight one aspect in people?

When you were younger and were asked what you wanted to be when you grew up, how did you respond? Did you respond, "I want to be known and make my mark on this world, not for my talents, abilities, or character, but because I chose to have a certain type of preference"? Or did you have more talent-driven ambitions, such as being a pharmacist, nurse, or doctor? Others may have desired to be an engineer or an athlete. Or maybe a firefighter, architect, or police officer? Or perhaps a baker, geologist, or business owner of your own making? At what point was the decision made to choose your "identity" to be based on one thought or one preference?

How has society capitalized on the concept of defining yourself based on a thought or preference? How is it that businesses now require continuing education or competencies to occur and be stored in personnel files for documentation regarding preference *training*? What about focusing on the safety of our patients and customers? Or our children? Or the safety of our country? Could infrastructure be an important thing to focus on instead? How about the importance of a standard of conduct in companies so employees are treated decently and are acknowledged for hard work and talent? How about analyzing the company's termination policies? How is it that businesses are forced to become more concerned about a thought or "preference" rather than if someone is skillfully qualified to perform their job description? How did this happen? Because I prefer to put my left shoe on before my right shoe, is this how I should choose to "identify" myself?

I believe I am of more value than labeling myself based on one thought of how I "prefer" to perform an action. Would a new competency be created that all employees would be mandated to perform based on which-shoe-first preference? More importantly, what can be done to refocus on priorities, and what would be the most efficient and productive manner of operation? Certainly, there must be a way that everyone can still be their own individual yet not "feel" a need to define themselves by a single element and then *force* their preferences into mandates, changing how businesses operate.

Why is there an increasing need to "identify" in *any* way in the first place? When did the change occur from logic and sound reasoning, which medical professionals excel at, to "feelings," which are unpredictable and unreliable? The "medical" healthcare of the past is evolving into "mental" healthcare despite the logical and scientific basis the medical field has derived from.

Employees and employers are being forced to actually *favor* people with a different thought or "preference." What does that have to do with work? What is the basis of how this relates to work productivity and successful accomplishment? What about innocent children who should focus on a playful childhood rather than on "preferences"? This pressure has nothing to do with the child and everything to do with adults forcing the idea upon them. What is the reason for encouraging children, whose minds are not fully developed, to have to "identify" themselves? As a matter of fact, on average, as you already know, the brain is not fully developed until approximately age twenty-five. Is it logical to ignore this fact?

Why would businesses be forced to focus on how a person "identifies" rather than on the abilities of the employees? What does the workplace, or any place of business or public gathering, have to do with a focused look at a preference? For example, it is contradictory to have sexual harassment competencies yet force everyone to focus on their "sexual identity" and give special consideration to people who choose to make that the focus of their being rather than anything work-, skill-, or character-related. Will they eventually give special consideration to people who prefer to put a shoe on their left foot first and develop competencies for this "preference"?

The other day, I called a new eye doctor to schedule an appointment for what I considered a concern for my eyes. There was a very nice woman on the other end of the line. She asked logical questions and gathered important information. Then she asked me, "How do you identify?" Identify?

I said, "Well, I am a person noticing some blurriness and potentially even some double vision."

That wasn't the information she was looking for. I was seeking help with my vision, yet she wanted to discuss my view of *sexual* preference. How is this even logical? Was her knowledge of my views going to better help my vision? Would it serve to verify the health of my eyes? Should I have mentioned my left-foot-first shoe preference? What is the basis or logic for asking this question? Where does it ultimately stem from? And why is society laying down a red carpet to oblige this need for labeling you with an "identity"? Speaking from a critical thinking point of view, it defied logic.

*Potential reasons someone might feel a need to distinctly
define themselves with a type of "identity"*

1. *Insecurity.* We all have had some form of insecurity in our
    lives. It is part of our human nature. What are some that
    come to mind that you endured yet overcame? Was it a long
    process? How did you strategically overcome this obstacle?
    Did you use reason and logic to make sense of the obstacle?
    Are there any insecurities you can think of that still linger?
    How does a sense of insecurity present itself to you? How
    do you respond to the situation when you are made aware
    of it? Who or what are the potential sources of the insecu-
    rity? Is it generally from words that were spoken or from
    an event that may or may not have happened? What are
    other alternatives to try to work through insecurities and
    bring them to a resolution? Have you ever looked at the
    opposing side of the insecurity, if there is one? How could
    seeing an alternate version affect your perspective? What
    type of research did you perform to understand the source
    of the problem? How can you research authentically and
    factually while showing no emotional bias? Did you resolve
    it within your own means? Could there be some underly-
    ing insecurity causing the desire to express to the world
    a particular way to define yourself? What are the talents
    and abilities that you have been blessed with? How are you
    utilizing these skills productively in your life? What if you
    defined yourself based on a different aspect? How many
    attributes can you think of to define yourself? What would
    change if you chose a different one? What if you placed
    all definitions aside and allowed yourself to be considered
    a worthy individual who is good just as you are without a
    label? Discover the source of the insecurity using reason
    and logic. Make an intentional effort to uncover the source
    and use skills and any necessary help to work through and
    heal your insecurity, leaving you better able to enjoy a con-
    tented and fulfilled life.

2. *Herd mentality.* Many things are easier when you are in the comfort and security of a group. As mentioned earlier, there is strength in numbers. Often, there is a combined sharing of different perspectives, leading to productive solutions. As many come together with the same "desire" to *feel* accepted, it becomes easier to build strength in almost anything. Is the idea of acceptance from like-minded people causing more people to join a "bandwagon"? Is there comfort or a *feeling* of acceptance if you join in and align with others? Have you taken the time to think about why this has happened? Is there a sense of obligation while in the presence of the group? Are you permitted to critically think for yourself and reach your own conclusions without fear of reprisal of some sort? Sometimes in a group setting, people can slip into the role of a follower, losing their *true* identity as an individual. Do you allow others to think for themselves without prejudice, respecting potentially different views? Are you able to still be yourself, despite potential persuasion, because of a group mentality? Are you highlighting your best characteristic? What are some of your other characteristics? Or are you just following a crowd? Do you find security under the umbrella of a group? What do you see as the benefit derived from a group? Would there be a bigger benefit from being away from the influence of the group? How would this be different? What factors have you considered in reaching your conclusions? Is there a chance you have given up your individual freedom for conformity?

3. *Desire for attention.* It can be difficult always to be in the background or to be shy and *feel* like you are unnoticed. Everyone appreciates at least a little attention at some point. Perhaps the desire to be seen and recognized for something is a reason for taking a defined outlook on life. Do you want to be noticed by people and catch their attention? Whom would you like to be noticed by? Have you thought about different captivating ways to reach people? In what

ways have you tried to get involved? What other ways can you reach out and be noticed based on your abilities or accomplishments? What would be the benefit of this? How are you impacted when you are noticed? How about when you are not noticed? Is this the best decision you reached in regard to gaining some form of attention? What other forms of attention might be endearing? What may have happened in your past that led you to be subdued? What type of research might support the idea of drawing attention to yourself? Is defining yourself by choosing an "identity" satisfying your desire? If so, in what ways does this further your goals or values? What other attributes, characteristics, or actions might there be to be noticed? What type of attention might win the hearts of people without biasing others?

4. *Peer pressure.* Peer pressure is a powerful force everyone has probably experienced at one point or another in their lives. While it could be a positive or negative force, it is generally considered negative as it implies that your ability or opportunity to control your own decisions is actually influenced and *controlled by* someone else. Are you being pressured to act in a certain way? Who might be putting unwarranted pressure on you? What would the basis for this pressure be? Who would benefit from following suit with this pressure? Do you put pressure on yourself to act or be a certain way? Has someone allowed you to feel the need to take a stand and narrow the way in which you see yourself? Was there a time in your life when you clearly felt pressured by your peers? What were the surrounding circumstances? How did you respond to this situation? What are other ways you could have responded to the situation? Were you able to remain strong and *not* allow yourself to be persuaded by others? What other thoughts do you have about peer pressure? Learn how to recognize if someone is attempting to snatch your power away from you by pressuring you to think or act like them. Be aware at all times of the possibil-

ity of someone or something trying to *take control* of your freedom and individuality. It can happen in the subtlest of ways. Make an effort to see the situation from an opposing perspective, and then evaluate your information in an unbiased manner. Question and discover more about the motives or agendas of others in persuasive situations. Ask yourself who benefits from giving up your control. Then, draw your own independent conclusions without pressure from others.

5. *Emotionally charged.* It can be very difficult to think straight when those around you are emotionally charged. It may even be a little or a lot intimidating! How about the way you make decisions when *your* emotions are running on the high side? What do you do to calm down and critically think about the situation? Has a highly emotional state, either yours or someone else's, been the driving force behind *feeling* the desire to label yourself? Emotions can be powerful, yet they may cloud the ability to think rationally. It is not hard to get caught up in an emotionally driven cause or event. The influence can be formidable, as emotion may lead to unpredictability. What is the basis for your decision-making choices? How do emotions typically affect you? Can you think of a time when emotions clouded your decisions? What were the results of the situation? Who was involved, and who benefitted from the emotional stance? How about a time when you overcame an emotional situation by resolving it rationally? What steps did you take for this to occur? Are there other areas in your life driven by emotions? How do you evaluate and handle emotional situations? What is your particular way to unwind or cope when emotions are involved? What is your source of replenishing calmness in your immediate environment? How can you gain more control over your emotions?

6. *Hurt.* We have *all* been hurt in one way or another in our lifetimes. *No one* leaves this world unscathed. It is prob-

ably almost *guaranteed* that we will be hurt again. The way pain is afflicted is different for every person. Yet, not everyone *feels* the need to react publicly. Some call it *oppression* and seek revenge. Others focus on healing themselves and building stronger, empowering, and uplifting qualities within themselves, transforming their negative energy into positive vibrations and pouring it out toward successful personal or professional development. How do you handle mentally painful situations that occurred through no fault of your own? How about physically painful situations? How about a hurtful situation you may have caused, even if it was by accident? Do you let a *historically* painful event, unexperienced by you personally, *control you* and how you respond today? Do you let the pain *define* who you are and how you act or react? How would lashing out solve anything? Who benefits from being *reactive* rather than *proactive*? Do you understand that *everyone* has had some form of pain in their lives, not simply you? While it is very unfortunate that you are hurting, what are better methods to *heal, remove* the pain, and *move forward peacefully* rather than allow yourself to be *controlled* by it? A *choice* can be made to find the source of the pain, address it in a healthy, positive, and joy-filled way, and alleviate the hurt permanently! Have you taken the time to see things from an opposing perspective? Do you choose to be influenced by the pressure of others, or are you *unwilling* to act based on emotion and pressure? How do you evaluate the source of the hurt? What methods do you undergo to heal? How can you alter any negative responses regarding the source of the pain? What do you know about the source of the pain? Who or what is the cause? What is your desired outcome of choosing an "identity" derived from a hurt? Does this permanently resolve the problem without harming or focusing on anyone else in the process, allowing contentment and productivity to prevail? What outcome do you extrapolate from a certain tag? Are you able to let go of bitterness and forgive? Or do you hold on to the bitterness, let it *control* you, and use it to inflame someone else? In what ways can you *choose* to let go of the hurt and gain your control back? Think of numerous methods that involve your healing *without* inflicting further hurt upon anyone else. In my book, *Success Is Ele-MENTAL*, this is what I call *"successfully revenged."* All of the energy and passion from the painful event is focused on your ability to become *massively successful* and highly prosperous while *removing* the source of hurt from your mind. You are taught how to reprogram your mind to automatically focus on success and positive and empowering energy. As long as you let hurtful sources *control* your mind and continue to focus on them, they continue to win no matter what you do. Let them go *completely* and focus on leading a successful, bitter-free, and joyful life, unaffected by the negativity of others or by the thoughts from the past. How would focusing on healing and building positive and fruitful energy in your own life change your perspective? How would your health and outlook benefit from healing your heart *and* mind? Has your method of resolving a hurtful event ever involved meditation or prayer? Who is a close friend who will listen without prejudice? How can you *be* this kind of friend to others? How can you not let pain define and control you? Consider ways you can hold onto your freedom to think as an individual rather than conform to the guise of others.

7. *Sensitized.* Many things and people are becoming increasingly sensitized today. People *choose* to allow their *feelings* to be hurt at the slightest sign of discomfort. It appears people lately have been taking things quite personally and becoming "offended" at the slightest verbiage. How are you *sensitized* by things people say? What can you do not to allow cruel words to affect you personally? Being "offended" is a *choice.* The one "offended" has now *made it* their problem. How can you evaluate the truth or falsehood of the words others say? Perhaps the other person is hurting and does

not know how to process their feelings, so they *take it out* on you. How can you be aware when this occurs? What can you do to instinctively "critically think" about what they have just said and done so you can reveal the truth behind the words or the event? Do you become *emotional* if things aren't exactly as you would like them to be? Or are you able to be *tolerant* and forgiving? How can you become more tolerant and forgiving? How could you benefit from becoming this way? Do you stop and think about both sides of a situation? Or are you quick to react, taking things personally? Or respond like water off a duck's back, sensing there is a deeper, underlying issue with the *other* person, and the problem is actually *their* problem? How can you become more confident and able to think critically rather than *feeling* or actually becoming sensitized? Perhaps you could focus on enjoying the world a little more and taking people's actions a little less seriously. How skilled are you at practicing patience and extending grace to others? These can both be *very* challenging skills to perform! Yet both are *extremely admirable* qualities to encompass. Both would be incredible qualities to "identify" as if you must identify at all. Would you like patience, grace, and forgiveness extended to you when you were at fault or in need of compassion? Realize that "feelings" are a choice you make based on the programming of your thoughts. They do not define you, nor is it wise to base your actions on them. They are *unreliable* and *subject to change circumstantially*. Reprogram your mind with solid, objective thoughts that you choose, aligned with your values, and embed them in your mind with your individually selected program as defined in *Elevate Your Mind to Success*. Allow this programming to produce automatic, *logical* responses that parallel your belief system and provide contentment in your daily life. You will never regret a decision made based on logic. However, a decision based on "feelings" is subject to change based on the situation and can lead to long-lasting regret.

8. *To counter shame or guilt.* We have all done things in life that we may feel shameful for or maybe ridden with guilt. I certainly hope I am not just speaking for myself! There are so many life lessons to be learned. Some people (like me) generally end up learning the hard way! Think of a time or event when you felt ashamed of something you did or said. How about when you felt guilty? How did you respond or react during any of these circumstances? Would you react the same way today if another similar situation occurred? How might you respond differently? Have you ever let guilt or shame influence you to do something bold to overcome the negative feelings attached? How can you critically think about the basis of guilt or shame in an unbiased manner? Is there a link between past treatment you endured and a new desire to define yourself? How can this be an effective way to resolve those *feelings*? What other alternatives can you think of to create a new vision of an unfortunate occurrence? How can you heal feelings of guilt or shame so you can react based on *logic* and *reason* rather than on emotion? How would this be beneficial? Consider the opposing sides of healing versus reacting. Does an attempt to change other people's perspectives change how you view yourself? How are you affected by how others see you? Think about ways to productively heal unfavorable *feelings* from the past and move forward peacefully and *logically* without pressure to react.

9. *Pride.* Pride is said to be one of the most destructive and dangerous qualities. There is a good pride and a sinful pride. It is good to be proud of your children or perhaps even your accomplishments or abilities. There is a positive and upbeat implication attached to this type of pride, affecting others favorably. The other type of pride carries with it negativity and destructive properties. It is evil-based and *self-serving*. This type of pride is restrictive, conde-

scending, and poisonous, and it carries with it the potential or even the desire to hurt someone else or prove something. To understand which sense of pride is in effect, ask yourself critical thinking questions. What or who is the source of your pride? What type of energy is attached to the pride: negative or positive vibrations? What is the desired outcome in response to the pride? Does it stem from a place of hurt and pain or a place of joy, contentment, and encouragement? What is the reason for the pride? What is your source of information in the circumstance? Is the intent either to help someone or hurt someone? Set aside your own bias and evaluate the claim. Look at it from different viewpoints. What conclusions do you draw based on the information you collected? What do you think is going on? What information is most important in your determination? How do you know you have all the information? What is your direction in the position you have chosen? How might the stance you are taking affect other people? How do you intend for them to be affected? Analyze if your motives are present and determine your reason for engaging them. Could pride be clouding your judgment in any way? How do you determine the answer to that? If unhealthy pride is involved, how can you address these "feelings" and reprogram your thoughts to positive and uplifting ones? Beware of any prideful tendencies and use logic to reason the circumstances involved.

Take some time to think critically about the source of the desire to have a defined identity or perhaps consider why someone else might be led to this desire. What seems to be the underlying reason for this happening? What or who has led to this decision? What is the expected or at least desired outcome? What are the benefits that are linked to having a label? What are the benefits without it? How can you independently establish this decision without influence from anyone else? How would you describe the emotion attached to the decision for someone to define themselves? How can you reevaluate the situation, take your personal bias out, and see things from other vantage points? Is the decision full of positive or negative energy? How can you make it all positively energy-based? What is it that you truly want to be known for? Do you want to be defined by a thought? By an action? Or what about by an ability? Or perhaps by an act of service to others? How would you like your obituary to read if available to be seen for generations to come? What words of description would you like to be on your tombstone engraved permanently? Is there still a desire to "identify" as anything? Have you thought of other qualities you possess that would define you better, leaving you feeling uplifted or enlightened? Critically think about the idea of "identifying" yourself. Think of the pros, cons, and reasons involved. Also, think about why you would choose a certain tag. Consider your answers, opposing answers, and other alternatives from an unbiased perspective. Where does this lead your thoughts?

> *There will always be someone willing to hurt you, put you down,*
> *gossip about you, belittle your accomplishments and judge your soul.*
> *It is a fact that we all must face. However, if you realize that God*
> *is a best friend that stands beside you when others cast stones you*
> *will never be afraid, never feel worthless and never feel alone.*
> —Shannon Alder

> *There are moments when troubles enter our lives and we can do*
> *nothing to avoid them. But they are there for a reason. Only when*
> *we have overcome them will we understand why they were there.*
> —Paulo Coelho

> *Every second you dwell on the past you steal from your*
> *future. Every minute you spend focusing on your problems*
> *you take away from finding your solutions.*
> —Robin Sharma

> *I've learned that people will forget what you said, people will forget*
> *what you did, but people will never forget how you made them feel.*
> —Maya Angelou

Let your hopes, not your hurts, shape your future.
—Robert H. Schuller

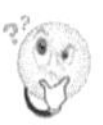

Reflect

1. Are you a person who finds it necessary to "define" yourself? If so, how do you define yourself? Do you know other people who feel this need?
2. What is the basis or driving factor that leads to this position? Is there positive or negative energy involved?
3. Do you ever allow *feelings* to affect your decisions? In what ways can feelings be unreliable?
4. How do you allow "logic" and "reasoning" to affect your decisions?
5. How have your past events influenced who you are at this very moment?
6. Think about how you would like to be thought of in years to come. Is your current stance in line with your desired legacy? Are there any changes you would like to make?
7. Write what you would like your obituary to say. What *is* your desired legacy? What steps do you need to take to lay the foundation for this legacy?

CHAPTER 12

Who's to Blame?

Have you noticed there is more finger-pointing in the world around you today than ever before? Very few, or perhaps almost none, seem to be at fault for all the issues around you, professionally as well as personally, yet everyone is blaming *everyone else* as the one at fault. Taking responsibility for one's own actions is becoming a rare occurrence, yet it is a highly regarded and impressive attribute to encompass. Blame is a claim that someone other than yourself is responsible for a certain act, cause, situation, or, lately, even a *feeling* one experiences. There are even *movements* occurring based on the *belief* that "it" was someone else's fault. If you have ever met or owned your own teenager, you know exactly about the blame game. Nothing is ever their fault! But it is time to critically think about the concept of partaking in this same action of blaming others and look at the *actual* source leading to this potential action.

I once worked for a company run by an unqualified management staff who promoted employees to a higher rank based on whoever was willing to accept the position when an opening presented itself. My boss, as a matter of fact, had a criminal record and had never held a management position before. Still, she was the only one at the time who was willing and had the required license available, so she received the position and title with no additional management skill training.

In this same company, all employees were required to hold a current CPR certification, yet the word around the workplace was that if something happened to a patient, you were not permitted to perform CPR on them. Using my critical thinking skills, I asked myself, *Why would we be required to hold an active certification if we were not permitted to use the skills to potentially save a life?* It appeared to be an illogical process. So, I asked around random employees and consistently received the same response from *every* one of them: "I don't know." I then contacted the head of the education department and asked this very same question. I received a disappointing, surprising, and extremely unhelpful response. Quite defensively, she asked, "Where did you hear that? Who said this? Give me a specific name right now. Who was it?"

Wow. Such a defensive stance was taken that in no way helped find a resolution to the question I had presented. How would finding out "who" (which was actually *everyone* I had asked) help bring the issue closer to resolution? How would giving the names of those who did not know the answer provide an answer to whether or not the act of CPR was permitted to occur? What was the premise of asking these questions? Was there a deficiency in the education department in relaying critical information? Was the response a personal agenda? Why was this person seeking a name to blame rather than focusing on a solution? How would knowing a name in which to place blame begin the process of educating the employees on a procedure that had been confusing the *entire* staff for what appeared to be a *very* long time?

Reasons people choose to blame others

1. *Fear.* Fear covers a large array of territory, including some of the points that follow. *False-events-appearing-real* is a crippling *feeling* that causes people to do or say unfortunate or unnecessary things. What is fear? Is there fear of reprisal for not performing the duties of a job? Fear of *feeling* inadequate? Where does the fear stem from? What is the worst-case scenario if the fear comes to fruition? Recalling that

fear is something that has *not actually happened*, what are possible situations that may occur? How likely are they to occur? What evaluation can be performed to shed light on alternatives? Who is involved with this fear? What result is desired from choosing to blame others in a situation based on fear? What ways could be chosen to be more productive? What if the choice could be made to focus on a *solution* rather than on fear? What could this possibly hurt? Or could it be helpful? How could the fear be overcome? What methods are currently being used? How can all bias be taken out of a scenario to find a productive solution rather than blame someone? What if the situation was in reverse? How would you handle unwarranted blame because of fear being placed on you? How can you create a situation with positive energy where it becomes instinctive to seek solutions rather than choose a defensive stance? How could this improve the environment around you? How would this change your workplace atmosphere? What are ways you can identify fears, reason them out, and eliminate them?

2. *Guilt.* Guilt may leave an empty and anxious *feeling* looming inside. Guilt could lead to blaming someone else for something that occurred with the possible intent of temporarily relieving the anxiety. What is the basis of the guilt? Where does it stem from? What are the circumstances that surround the situation? How can the guilt be resolved in an unbiased way within your own means? What have you learned from the situation? How would you respond differently next time? What would the premise be of blaming someone else for an issue because of feelings of guilt? What are other ways that the situation could be dealt with without blaming someone else? What is the truth in the situation? How do you handle *feelings* of guilt? Is there a need to step back and resolve any situations of guilt? How has this shaped your decisions? How can logic and reasoning be utilized in reframing guilt? What conclusions can you draw for an effective resolution?

3. *Pride.* As discussed in the previous chapter, could the "hurtful" type of pride be a reason for choosing to blame someone else? What are the surrounding circumstances of pride? How did the situation of blame arise? What are some alternate ways to respond rather than blaming someone else? Who is involved in the circumstance involving pride? What is a response that could lead to a productive outcome? Evaluate the situation. What are all of the circumstances that have led to the response? How did the response fit the evaluated information? What is the desired outcome of the reaction? How can pride be addressed to resolve the negative feelings attached to it? Often, a temporary "good" feeling will still leave you empty or hurting inside once again, as the issue itself has not been resolved, such as it would be if the feelings were reframed and properly healed. How can you decipher the source of the pride? How can you heal negative feelings so there is a lasting resolution rather than a temporary Band-Aid put on the problem? What if you tried to *resolve* the source to heal rather than react and rebuke?

4. *Hurt.* Hurt can lead to a multitude of responses, one of which can be "lashing out" and blaming someone else. Has someone who was hurting ever "lashed out" and blamed you for something? How did you handle this situation? Was this ever a pathway you chose? Who was involved in this interaction? How did this resolve the issue? Have you ever allowed hurt to be a reason to blame someone for something? How do you rationalize this decision? What type of research was performed before you made this decision? What is the basis of the decision? What other options for resolution are there? How could you respond differently? What would happen if you resolved the hurt feelings first? What alternative approaches could you take to handle the situation? Have you ever had a successful outcome by blaming someone else? Have you viewed the situation from an opposing perspective? How did you choose the person

you picked to blame? How did they hurt you? How will you *logically* move past the hurt?

5. *Insecurity.* Have you ever blamed someone because of an insecurity you had or have? Has anyone ever blamed you because of the insecurity *they* had? Who was involved in the circumstance? What role did they play? What were the circumstances that led to this decision? What research did you perform to reach the decision on which to act? What are some alternative choices that could've been made? What is the insecurity? How has this affected your life? What steps have you taken in an attempt to eliminate the insecurity? How did you evaluate the steps it would take? Who could help with the source of the insecurity? How did you justify your responses? Would you choose a different way to respond? How has insecurity caused you to respond in other circumstances? Have you been able to find a way to take control of the insecurity? How will you logically resolve the insecurity?

6. *Peer pressure.* Peer pressure is a consistent and repetitious force that will always be a contention in our lives. Have you ever allowed pressure from someone else to cause you to blame another person for something? Have you ever pressured someone else in the same way? How did you reach the decision to do this? Who was involved in the circumstance? Were they actually guilty or not? How did you respond when the decision was made? What would have been an alternative way to respond? How often do you hand over control to someone else because of pressure? How can you be more aware when you are being pressured and step back to critically think about the situation from an unbiased perspective? Have you ever been the recipient of blame because of peer pressure? How was it resolved? How can you overcome the influence of someone else and make your own decisions?

7. *Irresponsibility.* Everyone has been brought up differently and under differing circumstances. What were your cir-

cumstances like? What type of emphasis was placed on being responsible? Who was involved in developing your character? How much emphasis was placed on this development? Have you ever blamed someone to "dodge" responsibility? What are ways in which this could happen? How could it be prevented? What are ways you can develop the character quality of being responsible? How can you take responsibility for your actions? How are others affected if you aren't responsible for your actions? What benefits are involved in being responsible? What consequences might occur if you did not take responsibility for your actions? How do the people who surround you respond when the responsibility is theirs? What would happen if you made this a steadfast quality in your life? What could the benefits be?

8. *Unaccountability.* Have you ever been in a situation where someone was not accountable for their actions, and it negatively affected you? Who was involved? How did you respond? What were the consequences? Has there been a time when you were not accountable for your actions? Have you ever blamed someone when the accountability was actually yours to admit? What were the circumstances surrounding this event? Who was involved? How was the recipient affected by your decision? What are other ways you could have responded? What are some possible different outcomes? How can you evaluate each of these scenarios? How could the situation have been handled better? How can you be more accountable for your actions and your words? It's important to be accountable for yourself. It takes integrity and an authentic person to accept accountability for *all* of the actions they choose. How can you program this quality into your mind so it becomes an instinctive response?

9. *Reputation.* Sometimes, to spare a reputation, people may choose to blame someone else for something they have done. Has this ever happened to you? Has someone ever blamed

you for something they did to protect their reputation? How did you handle the situation? Have you ever blamed someone else for something to protect *your* reputation? In either case, what was the outcome? Who was involved in the blame? What are some better alternatives regarding how the situation could have been addressed? How do you wish you had responded? In what ways could the result be positive for both sides? How did you find yourself in this predicament to begin with? How was the other person affected? In what ways can you avoid a future occurrence like this? What have you learned about the situation?

10. *Uneducated or uninformed.* A lack of education can be an element leading to blame. Have you ever been blamed by someone who didn't fully understand a situation? How about the reverse circumstance? Have you ever accused someone else before you had all of the facts? How did you expect the outcome to play out? How did it actually turn out? Who was involved in this circumstance? What choices could you have made differently? How many options did you entertain before you made your decision on how you responded? How much and what kind of research did you do in preparation for your action? How could you become better informed about the situation? What would you change about your responses? How can you use this information for future situations? Has education, or lack thereof, been a problem before in making decisions? How do you stay up to date with information? Do you gather all the facts from your side and the opposing side before you come to a conclusion? How can you program this type of thinking into your mind for instinctive responses?

11. *Personality types.* People with different personality types can choose certain and almost predictable responses. Narcissists, for example, are notorious for blaming anyone in their pathway for anything they can think of. They are rarely, if ever, accountable for anything. It seems they are *never* wrong about anything in their eyes. Other toxic per-

sonality types respond the same way. Be aware of whom you are involved with and the potential for blame against you that may occur. How could a blame scenario with toxic personality types be avoided? What steps can you take to protect yourself? How much do you know about toxic personality types? Do you have one of these personalities? How would you respond in either case? How can you focus on the facts at hand and allow them to be the focus of the responses using an unbiased perspective? What education might be helpful to learn more about this topic? How do you recognize this type of personality type?

12. *Shame.* Have you ever been on the receiving end of blame, involving shame felt by another person? How did you handle this situation? What were the surrounding circumstances? Has shame ever driven you to blame someone else for something? What would be the premise of this action? What would be the expected outcome of blaming someone else? How could it be avoided? What is the source of shame? How can that be resolved? How can the *feeling* of shame be identified, understood, and dealt with to resolution? In what ways can this be avoided in the future? What do you know about shame? How can you help someone else who *feels* a sense of shame? What information can be researched to deal with this *feeling* in a healthy way?

13. *Financial incentive.* Has a financial incentive, either profitable or costly, ever been a reason used to blame someone else? Has someone blamed you for something, with finances being the influencing factor of the blame? Money can be very influential. What are ways you could see money affecting people? How might the influence of money cause someone to place blame on someone else? What might be the expected outcome? How can you ensure money is never used as an excuse to blame someone else? What would be the benefits of securing a plan? Do you know anyone who blamed someone else because of money matters? How did the matter transpire? How could this have been better

handled? What are the possible outcomes for this person? What did you learn from this experience? *Follow the money.*

14. *Justification.* People are capable of many sorts of things in their pursuit to justify themselves or their actions. Has anyone ever blamed you for something for the sake of their justification? Have you ever blamed someone else to justify something? Who was involved? What was the premise of the need to justify? What was the expected outcome of blaming someone else? Was the desired result received? What other choices could have been made? How would a change in previous decisions change the outcome? What could be done differently? Was the issue that needed to be resolved ever properly accounted for? What can be learned from this situation?

Blame is more and more common in all facets of life. It is even occurring based on historical events that are not even in existence today. What might be the reasons someone would place blame because of something that occurred in the past? Consider how often people allow their *feelings* to control their actions. There is a *lack of self-control,* growing exponentially, in society today. How would a past event not brought on by people currently today be a reason to place fault on someone today? What reasoning is used to justify blame for events of the past in the current setting? How might this situation look to those who are being blamed that were also not in the past events? How are they, or are they not, really at fault? How would it look if the situation was evaluated from the opposing side? What evidence is there to link the people of today with the actions of the past? What is the expected outcome of the action of blaming? What is the premise of the action? What has led to this action? What can be learned from history? How does blaming a historical event on current events today change anything? Does erasing the past make the events not real anymore? Or did they still really happen? What are alternative ways to handle the situation? What is a more productive response that can lead to a supportive and favorable current or future perspective? How can this be positively applied to your lifestyle today? Are you able to learn and grow because of it? How can you resolve any potential negative feelings and transform the energy into positive and productive energy?

Blame is an ineffective way to resolve *any* situation. It is a defensive stance that is counterintuitive to a resolution. How can you find alternative ways to view a situation? What other methods can you think of to resolve hurt *feelings* because of a past or other painful situation? What are the reasons for taking it personally, even if you were *not* personally there? What might happen if you had enough courage to accept the choices you made in life and where you are right now? If you are not happy with the scenario, what productive and positive changes can you make in your life to improve your situation? Without focusing on anyone else and a need to blame someone, how can you find enjoyment in life? What are your gifts and talents? How can you use them in fun, useful, productive, and creative ways? What activities do you enjoy? What is something you have always desired to accomplish or succeed in? What would it take to pursue this dream? How can you learn more about accountability?

Take responsibility for your actions. Be confident in who you are and where you are. Learn to think for yourself without prejudice, focus on self-improvement, and make choices that lead to true and continuous joy rather than a *temporary* Band-Aid to happiness.

Blame may provide a brief sense of satisfaction as it "justifies" a hurt, but this *temporary* happiness is subject to circumstances. Band-Aids will fall off, exposing the wound once again, whereas no one can take your joy away. Joy is a *sustainable* state of contentedness based on faith, hope, and security regarding what is to come, *not* on a temporary past or current circumstantial event. Seek to *fill your life* with joy.

All blame is a waste of time. No matter how much fault you find with another, and regardless of how much you blame him, it will not change you. The only thing blame does is to keep the focus off you when you are looking for external reasons to explain your unhappiness or frustration. You may succeed in making another feel

guilty about something by blaming him, but you won't succeed in changing whatever it is about you that is making you unhappy.
—Wayne Dyer

You can either blame everybody else or you can take a look at yourself and determine where you can improve.
—Robert Kiyosaki

If you could kick the person in the pants responsible for most of your trouble, you wouldn't sit for a month.
—Theodore Roosevelt

You will never become who you want to be if you keep blaming everyone else for who you are now.
—John Spence

You can get discouraged many times, but you are not a failure until you begin to blame somebody else and stop trying.
—John Burroughs

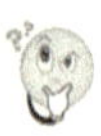

Reflect

1. Are you a person who finds it necessary to blame yourself or others? If so, what might be a better way to approach a situation?
2. What is the driving factor that may lead you to consider blaming someone else for something you did or experienced?
3. Think of someone you know who has a tendency to blame others. Now think of someone who takes on all of his or her own responsibility and is always accountable for their actions. Compare and contrast the differences between the two. What do you notice?

4. Looking at two or more different sides to a story, what might be a better approach to take in a difficult situation?
5. How have events in your past influenced how you perceive blame?
6. Think about how you would like to be thought of in years to come. Is your current view regarding blame in line with your desired legacy? Are there any changes you would like to make?
7. How can you be productive and incorporate the positive character qualities of responsibility and accountability into your programming?
8. Who can you share this outlook with who may benefit from its supportive nature?
9. Critically think about the concept of blame. What comes to mind?

CHAPTER 13

What Is Gaslighting?

Gaslighting *"is an insidious form of manipulation and psychological control."*[30] All of the following content of description included here is derived from this same source. This chapter is intended to introduce the topic of gaslighting, bring awareness of its common occurrence, and place it under critical thinking scrutiny. *"Victims of gaslighting are deliberately and systematically fed false information that leads them to question what they know to be true, often about themselves."*

Has any news media outlet ever executed anything like this before? How about politicians or other people in authority? Is there anyone you currently know who has personally experienced this? Or maybe you know someone who actually *is* a gaslighter? Generally speaking, the relationship starts out well in gaslighting and may even involve praise or sharing confidence to build a trusted bond. The more quickly the victim becomes enamored, the quicker the next phase of manipulation typically begins.

The gaslighter then proceeds to lie about simple little things, followed by an increasing volume and content of lies, which continues to grow. If the victim questions the gaslighter, the victim may be accused of lying as a way to protect the strategy of the gaslighter. Have *you* ever experienced this type of treatment? Have you seen it happen to someone dear to you? Did you recognize it as *gaslighting*, or did you not have a name for it at the time?

This type of treatment may become so intense and complex that the victim may end up *doubting their own memory, perception,* and even their *sanity.* It may even become difficult for them to see and recognize the truth. While the situation may start on a small level, the volume of misinformation may grow to be intense. Tactics are often employed to keep the victim engaged, such as showing some positive reinforcement to confuse the victim. Efforts may also be made to turn family and friends *against* this person by spreading lies to disassociate them from close bonds and create an "illusion of delusion."

The verbiage *gaslighting* originates from a 1938 play and film adaptation, *Gas Light.* Victims of gaslighting *"are targeted at the core of their being: their sense of identity and self-worth."*[31] What groups can you think of that may be, or already have been, susceptible to becoming targets of gaslighting manipulation by attacking their identity and self-worth? How are they lured in? Who is attempting to lure them in? What seems to be the reason for gaslighting them? What are the desired end results of gaslighting them? What could this change? Who benefits from gaslighting someone? What is the premise of targeting these people? Is the source overlooking, ignoring, or leaving out information that doesn't support its agenda? Is the source using unnecessary persuasive language to sway the victim's perception of the facts? The goal of this type of manipulation is to *attain power over* the victim through emotional, financial, or physical control.

What type of person is most susceptible to gaslighters?

1. Insecure
2. Lonely or alone, even a "loner"
3. Hurt or "oppressed"
4. Depressed or desperate
5. Involved in "group think" or "herd mentality"
6. Indecisive
7. Shy
8. Fearful or worrisome

9. Dependent
10. Has a follower mentality
11. Financially distraught
12. Circumstantially distraught
13. Mentally or physically distraught

Recognize the qualities mentioned previously as the most likely to fall prey to the guise of the gaslighter. The gaslighter will seek the most vulnerable, which are also the ones who will be most easily influenced. If you are in any of the categories mentioned, or perhaps you know of a patient, customer, or family member who may be vulnerable, be aware of this possibility and take extra precautions. Or better yet, develop an antidote to the previous issues, and embark on a journey of awareness and self-improvement strategies to strengthen confidence and increase your (already valuable) self-worth. More ideas can be found regarding further development of this skill set in my book *Success is Ele-MENTAL*.

Gaslighters may be dictators, leaders, politicians, news media outlets, domestic abusers, bosses, narcissists, or cult leaders, to name a few. The most effective gaslighters may be hard to detect, being better recognized by the *damage induced upon* the victim and his or her actions and mental state. *"Those who employ this tactic often have a personality disorder, narcissistic personality disorder, and psychopathy chief among them."*[32] They are often seen by the world one way and by the victim another. This also causes the victim concern for reaching out for help, fearing that they will not be believed. A gaslighter will typically repeat the behavior across several relationships. Keep in mind that gaslighters must have an *extreme* sense of insecurity, lack of compassion, and mental disability, as they believe controlling others is the *only* way they can succeed with their agenda. Yet, they are also sly, cunning, shrewd, and immoral. This is a dangerous combination.

A primary objective of gaslighters is to keep the victim *hooked*. If doubted or disagreed with, gaslighters may try to make *themselves* the ones being victimized. Gaslighters may make promises of changing and make claims to keep the victim holding on, although as soon as the victim agrees to continue, things likely revert back to how they were. Gaslighting can be psychologically devastating as it violates trust, alters the victim's view of people, and makes them suspicious of everyone close to them. A gaslighter also erodes a person's trust in themselves and causes them to forget what they once valued about themselves.

What is the difference between manipulation and gaslighting?

> *Manipulation is a key part of gaslighting, but manipulation is a fairly common tactic, and almost anyone is capable of employing it, while gaslighting, and gaslighters, are more rare. Gaslighting involves a pattern of abusive behaviors with the intent not just to influence someone, but to control them.*[33]

How has gaslighting crept into our society today? Do you see it in politics or news media outlets? How can you recognize when gaslighting is occurring? What might the agenda be for the one gaslighting? What could the underlying premise be? Who would benefit from gaslighting? What is deceitful in the approach of the source? How can you research to find more information? How can you decipher if a patient, customer, close friend, or family member is a victim? What factors would you look for? How could you help someone in this unfortunate situation? How would you identify a perpetrator? What factors would you look for in this case? Where are likely places where this tactic might be employed? How can you prevent someone from taking advantage of you?

Considering all of the information presented about gaslighting, can you see how this is another way certain people seek to *take away freedom* from others? Precious freedom in our society is under attack now more than ever. As each freedom is relinquished, another entity, such as the government, becomes stronger. Dwell upon the fact that because we are "the home of the brave," we became "the land of the free." Apply critical thinking methods to what our forefathers *sacrificed* to provide us with the very freedom we now enjoy. What would happen if freedom gave way to conformity, and we were all *under the control* of the "conformist"?

Learn how to identify the characteristics of a gaslighter and someone being abused by a gaslighter. Gaslighting is a cruel method of abusing powers of influence and manipulation to *control* and *undermine* someone else. Research many credible sources regarding this topic. Bring yourself to a clear understanding of what it is and how to easily identify when it occurs. Take time to critically think about the factors involved with this disorder, and consider ways, based on your own conclusions, to guard against this immoral misuse of power.

Narcissists are consumed with maintaining a shallow false self to others. They're emotionally crippled souls that are addicted to attention. Because of this, they use a multitude of games in order to receive adoration. Sadly, they are the most ungodly of God's creations because they don't show remorse for their actions, take steps to make amends or have empathy for others. They are morally bankrupt.
—Shannon L. Alder

Gaslighting is mind control to make victims doubt their reality.
—Tracy Malone

I first came across the term gaslighting in the context of abusive romantic partners, but it shows up in larger-scale relationships, too, like those between bosses and their employees, politicians and their supporters, spiritual leaders and their devotees. Across the board, gaslighting is a way of psychologically manipulating someone (or many people) such that they doubt their own reality, as a way to gain and maintain control.
—Amanda Montell

In terms of gaslighting, I define it as 'to implant false and/or distorted narratives that are specifically designed or formulated to manipulate a person into a destructive web of deception, loss

of control, and the surrender of personal freedom and beliefs of self-worth, self-value, self-esteem, and productivity.'
—Ross Rosenberg

Gaslighting is a subtle form of emotional manipulation that often results in the recipient doubting their own perception of reality and their sanity. In addition, gaslighting is a method of manipulation by toxic people to gain power over you. The worst part about gaslighting is that it undermines your self-worth to the point where you're second-guessing everything.
—Dana Arcuri

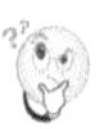

Reflect

1. Define the term *gaslighting*. How would you identify the characteristics of someone being abused by a gaslighter? How would you identify and define a perpetrator?
2. How has gaslighting affected you personally? Your patients? Your family? Your career or business?
3. How has gaslighting made its way into the political sector?
4. What is your biggest concern regarding gaslighting in positions of high authority?
5. How will you evaluate or research information concerning gaslighting without prejudice that you feel is concerning? How can you become better informed based on your own research?

CHAPTER 14

Conclusion

After much discussion and review of a vast number of ideas, thoughts, stories, and concepts, what have *you* concluded regarding *Medically Speaking, Who Connects Your Dots*? Did you determine whether or not *other* news media sources have taken on this role and taken over the connection for you? What about the Internet? Social media? CE sponsors or medical journals? The facility you work for? Or did you determine that *you* actually are in control of critical thinking and connecting your own dots by utilizing your *own* sound analysis and evaluation? Are there any changes or alterations you need or would like to make? Where will you be applying critical thinking methods? Who else could benefit from gaining an understanding of this process?

It is both fascinating and concerning to think about how many sources and which ones have programmed your mind since the day you were born. If not addressed, these other influences could continue to be the reason you respond as you do, sometimes challenging your very own values. Has the presented information caused you to think about the current programming of your mind?

In my previous book, *Elevate Your Mind to Success*, I lay the foundation for the basis of the preprogrammed mind and provide detailed thoughts, ideas, and suggestions on how to acknowledge your current programming and then remove, replace, or reframe your thoughts to align them with your current design of values and beliefs. This ties in with the focused and pragmatic ability to think critically, especially regarding sensitive or controversial matters you are faced with in your practice or your daily life in general. You must know who you are and what you believe in to properly reprogram your mind and to *instinctively* respond in ways that are *supportively* aligned with your values.

Be "on the lookout" for bias in the world that surrounds you, especially as it affects decisions that will affect your patients. You will find that it is *everywhere* you look, even in what we used to consider trusted and reliable medical resources. In some instances, it is tempting to succumb to the strategically "offensive" biases and respond with a just-as-emotional "defensive" reply. However, this could only further escalate the topic or situation at hand, flaring additional emotions in a senseless tizzy, all while defying logical thought. Or worse yet, it would be to concede to the information without verifying its validity. Take a step back, or maybe even two, and engage your *powerfully* effective critical thinking skills in an unprejudiced effort to draw on verified, extrapolated, and factual data, leading to logical insight.

In previous chapters, we discussed a few of the many ways your freedom is being snatched from you in plain sight. Some of these include biased major media outlets, erasing your history, censoring truth, and the brainwashing found in the educational school system. It is important to know how and why these things are happening. The rate of progression for these changes is astounding, and you can be certain that this movement will continue and expand as it does.

Learn how to discover unbiased yet factual research material and methods, and do your own analysis and evaluation. Use your critical thinking skills to evaluate opposing sides to bring more enlightenment to your analysis. Awareness is always the first step in any situation. Allow censorship and canceling to be *instant warnings* that something isn't right and that there is an attempt to hide the truth. Start to understand what and why things are progressing the way they are. The key here is to ascertain this information independently, free of prejudice.

The book continues by defining the vital method of critical thinking, the basis for this important action, and how to perform it properly. It is imperative to bring yourself to a full understanding of the methods and particulars of thinking in this manner. Critical thinking is a skill that *must* be practiced and mastered to contend with this vastly changing culture.

Taking an unbiased stance is necessary for the ability to comprehend *all* aspects of a situation and develop insight from *all* perspectives. Just as with the success of the Trojan horse in the city of Troy, there is always more clarity and a better position when you have access and insight into the opposing side's most vulnerable information. In addition, as more knowledge is gained, more doors may open with possibilities of an altered opinion or way of doing things.

Always be open to the possibility of absorbing new information that may lead to a fresh perspective you may have been previously unaware of. You may discover missing pieces to a story that changes your entire perspective. If you were not open to the possibility, you might be supporting something unintentional or unfavorable to your true beliefs.

The Milgram experiments, performed by Stanley Milgram, were brought forth and discussed, revealing human behavior regarding obedience while under authority. From these experiments, we learned that ordinary people might likely follow orders from an authority figure for one of many reasons, even to the extent of killing innocent human beings. Obedience to authority is ingrained in people to the degree that it has been preprogrammed into their minds. People are capable of acting as *agents* for another person's will.

Along with the guise of authority, many other factors are influential in "persuading" decision-making in people, which were discussed in previous chapters. Be aware of these factors and of how people can be easily influenced by others to do unethical or even unexplainable things while under their misguided pretenses.

Critical thinking methods were implored and practiced on a series of thought-provoking topics, including for potential reasons of feeling a need to identify and the common and growing stance today of placing blame on others rather than taking responsibility or being accountable for our actions. Both of these topics have appeared to "grow wings" of their own and have "taken flight." A source of this focus has been the use of numerous sources of propaganda.

Propaganda was defined, along with its intention, to control how you think and act. Propaganda relies on manipulation, and keys to successful manipulation were explored and discussed for thinking application. Discussion ensued regarding the book *Nineteen Eighty-Four* to exemplify the ingenious "premonition" of George Orwell regarding the potential result of manipulation, control, and brainwashing of people by authority figures with a self-serving agenda.

Finally, gaslighting, censorship, and cancel culture were defined and processed through the critical thinking method. Critical thinking is more important than *ever* before. Being skillfully adapted to this process helps awaken and potentially "immunize" you to the negative effects of manipulation, persuasion, and influence of powerful governing bodies that surround you, at least to a certain extent. It takes dedication, hard work, and a concentrated effort to master the skills of thinking critically.

Medically Speaking, Who Connects Your Dots has broken down the basic elements of critical thinking and has offered ideas, suggestions, examples, and questions to hone your skills to become a better and even instinctual critical thinker. By performing these skills, you will use logic to make informed, factual, and unbiased decisions, giving you an edge on your individuality and strength in your freedom against conformity.

The third-rate mind is only happy when it is thinking with the majority. A second-rate mind is only happy when it is thinking with the minority. A first-rate mind is only happy when it is thinking.
—A. A. Milne

The important thing is not to stop questioning.
Curiosity has its own reason for existing.
—Albert Einstein

*It is a mark of an educated mind to be able to
entertain a thought without accepting it.*

—Aristotle

*Critical thinking is not something you do once with
an issue and then drop it. It requires that we update
our knowledge as new information comes in.*

—Daniel Levitin

*The essence of the independent mind lies not in
what it thinks, but in how it thinks.*

—Christopher Hitchens

*Freethinkers are those who are willing to use their minds without
prejudice and without fearing to understand things that clash
with their own customs, privileges, or beliefs. This state of mind
is not common, but it is essential for critical thinking.*

—Leo Tolstoy

*To think incisively and to think for oneself is very difficult. We
are prone to let our mental life become invaded by legions of half-
truths, prejudices, and propaganda. At this point, I wonder whether
or not education is fulfilling its purpose. A great majority of the
so-called educated people do not think logically and scientifically.
Even the press, the classroom, the platforms, and the pulpit in
many instances do not give us objective and unbiased truths. To
save man from the morass of propaganda, in my opinion, is one of
the chief aims of education. Education must enable one to sift and
weigh evidence, to discern the true from the false, the real from the
unreal, and the facts from the fiction. The function of education,
therefore, is to teach one to think intensively and to think critically.*

—Dr. Martin Luther King Jr.

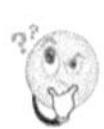

Reflect

1. Define the skill of critical thinking. Summarize its key elements. How will you apply these particular skills in your daily practice? Personal life?
2. How will you word questions so they are framed in an unbiased stance? Make a list of questions you will ask yourself when you employ the process of critical thinking.
3. What sources will you use to educate yourself further on critical thinking? How will you choose the sources? How will you validate the integrity of the sources?
4. What is your most significant insight or concern about the conclusions you came to regarding the manipulation surrounding you? What is the premise of your concern?
5. How has this information impacted the way you think?
6. How will you apply the information you've learned from this book to your daily life?
7. Who will you share this information with?

NOTES

1   Will Erstad, "6 Critical Thinking Skills You Need to Master Now," January 22, 2018, Accessed January 12, 2023, https://www.rasmussen.edu/student-experience/college-life/critical-thinking-skills-to-master-now/.
2   Turtles All the Way Down, free chapter, https://tinyurl.com/TurtlesBookChap1Eng.
3   Dr Robert Malone, "Do Not Comply," rwmalonemd.substack.com, Accessed September 8, 2023, https://rwmalonemd.substack.com/p/do-not-comply?r=jtms6&utm_campaign=post&utm_medium=email
4   "Milgram Experiment," Wikipedia, Accessed January 12, 2023, https://en.m.wikipedia.org/wiki/Milgram_experiment.
5   Liz Breazeale and Jenna Clayton, "When Was 1984 Written?", Study.com, December 02, 2021, Accessed January 16, 2023, https://study.com/academy/lesson/when-was-1984-written.html.
6   Will Erstad, "6 Critical Thinking Skills You Need to Master Now."
7   Edward Bernays, Propaganda (Ig Publishing, 2005), 168 pages.
8   John Hudson, "US Repeals Propaganda Ban, Spreads Government-Made News to Americans," foreignpolicy.com, July 14, 2013, Accessed March 15, 2023, https://foreignpolicy.com/2013/07/14/u-s-repeals-propaganda-ban-spreads-government-made-news-to-Americans/.
9   Turtles All the Way Down: Vaccine Science and Myth, all references, https://tinyurl.com/Turtles/BookEngRef.
10   Died Suddenly 2022 (Full Documentary), https://rumble.com/v1wcs7o-died-suddenly-2022-full-documentary.html.
11   Turtles All the Way Down.
12   FLCCC Alliance, Accessed February 26, 2023, https://covid19criticalcare.com.
13   FLCCC Alliance.
14   Andy Crump, The Journal of Antibiotics (2017), Accessed February 27, 2023.
15   FLCCC Alliance.
16   "17,000 Doctors and Scientists Signed a Treaty," Published January 21, 2021, Accessed February 26, 2023, https://guardiansofmedicalchoice.com/17000-signatures-on-physicians-declaration-global-covid-summit/ and https://doctorsandscientistsdeclaration.org.
17   Dr. Kelly Victory, Accessed February 27, 2023, https://earlycovidcare.org.

18 Dr. Drew, "'Foot-Long Blood Clots' from mRNA, Says Pathologists Dr. Ryan Cole w/ Dr. Kelly Victory – Ask Dr. Drew," Accessed February 26, 2023, COVID-19 vaccine, https://www.youtube.com/watch?v=2SLp6B_kkRI.

19 Dr. Ryan Cole, Accessed February 27, 2023, https://rcolemd.com.

20 Dr. Kelly Victory.

21 "Foot-Long Blood Clots."

22 Dr. Ryan Cole.

23 "17,000 Doctors and Scientists Signed a Treaty."

24 Peter McCullough, bibliography, Accessed February 26, 2023, https://orcid.org/0000-0002-0997-6355.

25 Dr. Frank Yap, MD, "Dr Peter McCullough: Fact Check and Debunked Theories," COVID Advisor, November 1, 2022, Accessed March 1, 2023, https://covid19.onedaymd.com/2021/12/dr-peter-mccullough-fact-check-and.html?m=1.

26 Robert W Malone, MD, "My Substack: Who Is Robert Malone?" Accessed March 1, 2023, rwmalonemd.com; https://www.rwmalonemd.com.

27 Died Suddenly 2022 (Full Documentary).

28 "Censorship," Wikipedia, 2023, Accessed January 23, 2023, https://en.m.wikipedia.org/wiki/Censorship.

29 "Cancel Culture," Wikipedia, 2023, Accessed January 23, 2023; https://en.m.wikipedis.org/wiki/Cancel_culture

30 "Gaslighting," Psychology Today, 2023, Accessed January 23, 2023, https://www.psychologytoday.com/us/basics/gaslighting.

31 "Gaslighting," Psychology Today.

32 "Gaslighting," Psychology Today.

33 "Gaslighting," Psychology Today.

CRITICAL THINKING QUESTIONS

To discover the truth, you must first ask the right questions.
—Jill Fandrich

Who is doing what?
What seems to be the reason for this happening?
What appears to be the desired end results?
How could they change?
What are the surrounding circumstances?
Whom does this benefit?
How does this affect you?
Does the source of this information appear to have an agenda?
What is the agenda?
Does the message have a bias?
Is the source overlooking, ignoring, or leaving out information that doesn't support its beliefs or claims?
Is there censoring involved for opposing views?
If so, why would this be?
Is the source using unnecessary or persuasive language to sway an audience's perception of a fact?
Is their funding involved?
Who is funding the source?
Is there a financial incentive involved?
How could this affect decisions?
How can you find reliable and credible resources?
How can you verify their credibility?
Is the information sourced or unsourced?

Is anything else being hidden?
What information is most relevant?
What other critical thoughts come to mind?
What do you think is going on?

Create your own questions:

1.

2.

3.

4.

5.

JOURNAL

—Jill Fandrich

Date:
Topic:

How could I have applied critical thinking to my interactions today?

What mistakes did I make?

How can I do it differently next time?

Where could I improve?

What did I do right?

156

What have I learned from this experience?

Other questions or thoughts?

JOURNAL

Great thinkers are note-*worthy.*

—Jill Fandrich

Date:
Topic:

How could I have applied critical thinking to my interactions today?

What mistakes did I make?

How can I do it differently next time?

Where could I improve?

What did I do right?

What have I learned from this experience?

Other questions or thoughts?

JOURNAL

Great thinkers are note-*worthy.*

—Jill Fandrich

Date:
Topic:

How could I have applied critical thinking to my interactions today?

What mistakes did I make?

How can I do it differently next time?

Where could I improve?

What did I do right?

What have I learned from this experience?

Other questions or thoughts?

JOURNAL

Great thinkers are note-*worthy.*

—Jill Fandrich

Date:
Topic:

How could I have applied critical thinking to my interactions today?

What mistakes did I make?

How can I do it differently next time?

Where could I improve?

What did I do right?

What have I learned from this experience?

Other questions or thoughts?

———————

JOURNAL

Great thinkers are note-*worthy.*

—Jill Fandrich

Date:
Topic:

How could I have applied critical thinking to my interactions today?

What mistakes did I make?

How can I do it differently next time?

Where could I improve?

What did I do right?

What have I learned from this experience?

Other questions or thoughts?

JOURNAL

Great thinkers are note-*worthy.*

—Jill Fandrich

Date:
Topic:

How could I have applied critical thinking to my interactions today?

What mistakes did I make?

How can I do it differently next time?

Where could I improve?

What did I do right?

What have I learned from this experience?

Other questions or thoughts?

JOURNAL

Great thinkers are note-*worthy.*

—Jill Fandrich

Date:
Topic:

How could I have applied critical thinking to my interactions today?

What mistakes did I make?

How can I do it differently next time?

Where could I improve?

What did I do right?

What have I learned from this experience?

Other questions or thoughts?

NOTES

NOTES

ABOUT THE AUTHOR

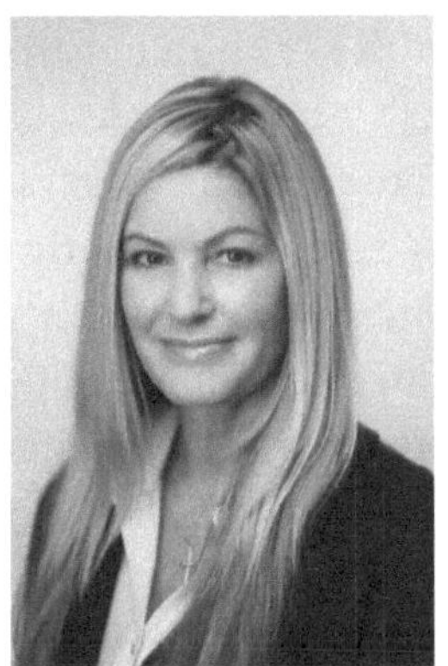

Jill Fandrich, PharmD, received her doctorate in pharmacy from Shenandoah University in Winchester, Virginia, and her degrees in chemistry and pharmacy from Westminster College and the University of Pittsburgh, respectively. During this time, she was a noted and accomplished public speaker, presenter and educator, diabetes care specialist, writer, artist, performer, director of a pharmacy, and media personality with a passion for helping people feel and live their best.

As an entrepreneur, Jill simultaneously became integrated into other endeavors of improving her community with house restoration and built corporations in the real estate and financial sectors, participating with other local entrepreneurs and businesses in joint cooperation of beautification.

Jill has most recently focused on her passion for writing to guide and encourage people and empower them to develop and discover their own unique and full potential. She is the author of *Elevate Your Mind to Success, Success Is Ele-MENTAL, Who Connects Your Dots?,*

COVID-19 Prevention, Parents: COVID-19 Prevention for Kids, and is a book reviewer and author of *A Book in Time Blog,* found at www. ABookinTime.net, where she educates, inspires, motivates, and energizes people to utilize their own unique skills and abilities to bring about the leader and success potential already located from within.

When not writing, Jill can be found spending time with friends and family; traveling; golfing; trading currencies; reading; running; walking; playing tennis; fixing, remodeling, or building things; being actively involved with her church; gardening; air-frying; or just puzzling on one of her hand-built puzzle boards.

Jill was born and raised in St. Marys, Pennsylvania, and has spent most of her life in Florida, currently residing in Fort Myers, Florida, where she continues to passionately write full-time regarding success strategies, leadership development, positive mind transformation, critical thinking, preventative medicine, and young adult, teen, and adult fiction novels.